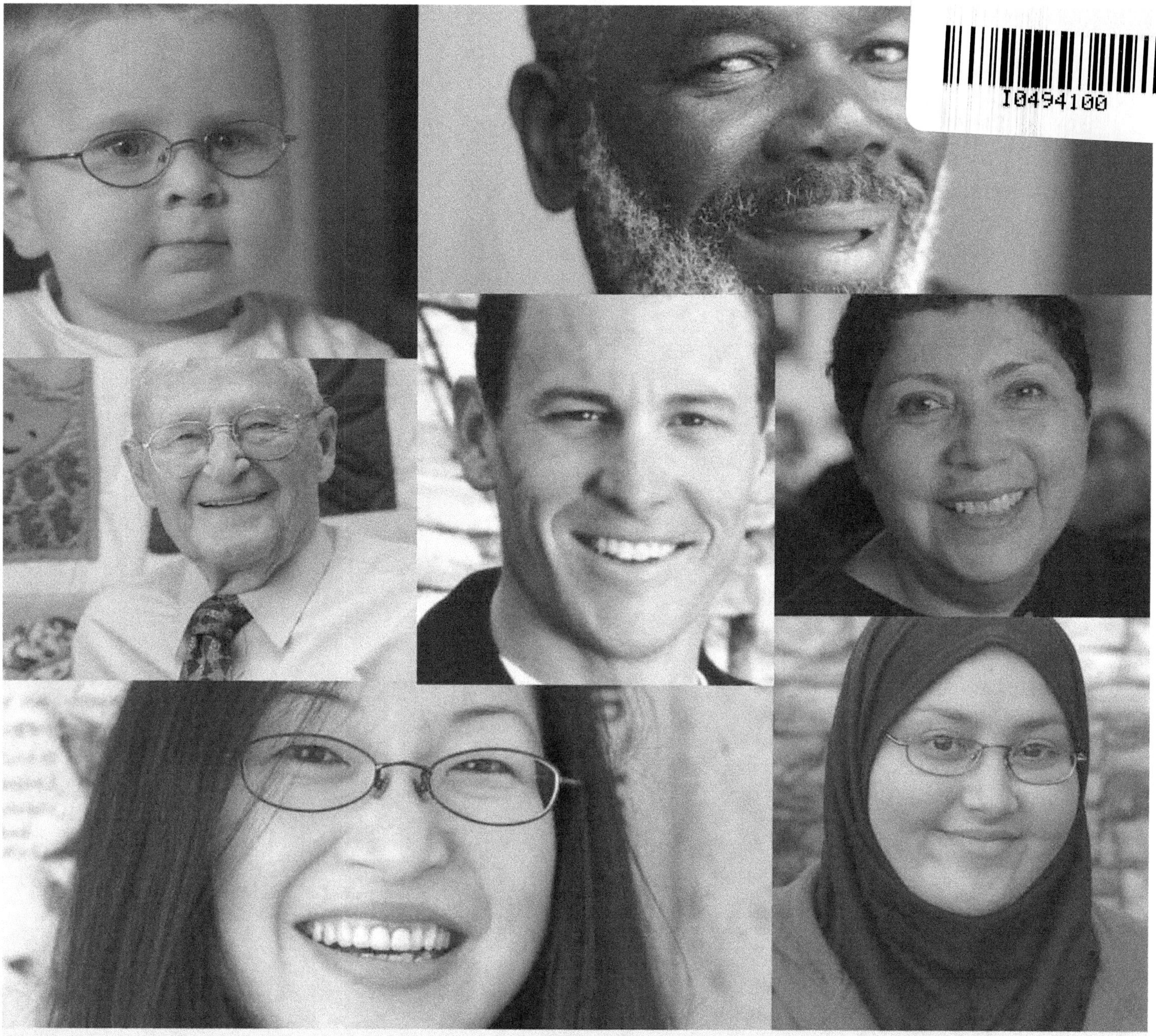

A National Action Plan for Cancer Survivorship: Advancing Public Health Strategies

DEPARTMENT OF HEALTH & HUMAN SERVICES·USA

CDC
SAFER·HEALTHIER·PEOPLE

LANCE ARMSTRONG FOUNDATION

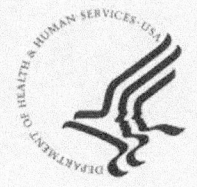

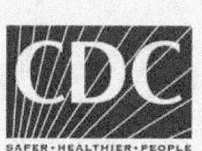

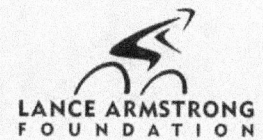

A National Action Plan for Cancer Survivorship:
Advancing Public Health Strategies

April 2004

This National Action Plan was developed to inform the general public, policy makers, survivors, providers, and others about cancer survivorship and public health. The National Action Plan was written to be read by audiences with varying levels of knowledge and awareness of cancer and/or survivorship issues. Each section has been written as a stand-alone component allowing the reader to focus on content specific to their interest. Therefore, some text is repeated to accommodate those who read selected sections at a time.

This publication was supported by Cooperative Agreement Number U57/CCU 623066-01 from the Centers for Disease Control and Prevention. Its contents are solely the responsibility of the authors and do not necessarily represent the official views of the Centers for Disease Control and Prevention, the Department of Health and Human Services, or the U.S. government.

CONTENTS

SPECIAL ACKNOWLEDGMENTS

We gratefully recognize the combined knowledge, effort, and commitment that our partners contributed to the completion of *A National Action Plan for Cancer Survivorship: Advancing Public Health Strategies*. We salute and thank the following partners who are leaders in the cancer survivorship field.

Cosponsors

Centers for Disease Control and Prevention
Lance Armstrong Foundation

Partners

Alaska Native Tribal Health Consortium
American Cancer Society
American Society of Clinical Oncology
Cancer Care Incorporated
Centers for Disease Control and Prevention
Children's Hospital of Los Angeles
Children's Hospital of Philadelphia
Children's Oncology Camp Foundation
Chronic Disease Directors
Congressman Roger Wicker's Office
Dana-Farber Cancer Institute
Fertile Hope, Inc.
Gilda's Club Worldwide
Institute for the Advancement of Social
  Work Research
Institute of Medicine
Intercultural Cancer Council
Maryland Cancer Plan
Michigan Department of Community Health
National Cancer Institute
National Coalition for Cancer Survivorship
National Hospice and Palliative Care
  Organization
National Institutes of Health
New York State Department of Health
North Carolina Division of Health and
  Human Services
Oklahoma State Department of Health

Oncology Nursing Society
Ovarian Cancer National Alliance
Presbyterian Hospital of Dallas
Patient Advocate Foundation
RAND Corporation
RTI International
Saint Jude Children's Research Hospital
Sisters Network, Incorporated
Sonnenschein Nath & Rosenthal
The Leukemia & Lymphoma Society
The National Center for Health Promotion
The Susan G. Komen Breast
  Cancer Foundation
The Unbroken Circle
Texas Cancer Council
Texas Department of Health
Ulman Cancer Fund for Young Adults
University of Texas Medical Branch
  School of Nursing
University of Minnesota
University of Pennsylvania Abramson
  Cancer Center
University of Rochester
University of Texas, M.D. Anderson
  Cancer Center
University of Texas Southwestern
  Medical Center
United States Conference of Mayors

INDEX OF ACRONYMS

ACS	American Cancer Society
BRFSS	Behavioral Risk Factor Surveillance System
CCC	Comprehensive Cancer Control
CDC	Centers for Disease Control and Prevention
CIS	Cancer Information Service
IOM	Institute of Medicine
LAF	Lance Armstrong Foundation
NAAP	National Arthritis Action Plan
NCCS	National Coalition for Cancer Survivorship
NCI	National Cancer Institute
NHIS	National Health Interview Survey
NIH	National Institutes of Health
NPCR	National Program of Cancer Registries
PHFSC	Public Health Functions Steering Committee
SEER	Surveillance, Epidemiology, and End Results
USDHHS	U.S. Department of Health and Human Services

EXECUTIVE SUMMARY

The Facts

Cancer is the second leading cause of death among adults in the United States and affects an estimated 1 in 3 individuals in their lifetime, either through their own diagnosis or that of a loved one (ACS, 2003). Increasing innovations in medical technology have led to earlier diagnoses and improved treatment of many cancers, resulting in more people diagnosed with cancer surviving each year. Currently, approximately 62% of cancer survivors are expected to live at least 5 years after diagnosis (ACS, 2003). As of January 2000, there were approximately 9.6 million cancer survivors in the United States (NCI, 2003a). This estimate includes people diagnosed with cancer but does not include others affected by a diagnosis, such as family members and friends.

The Challenge

Public health programs address the prevention and control of health problems affecting large groups of people. Although many public health initiatives address early detection, prevention, and control of cancer, public health is new to the cancer survivorship arena. Throughout this National Action Plan, the term "cancer survivors" refers to those people who have been diagnosed with cancer and the people in their lives who are affected by their diagnosis, including family members, friends, and caregivers. Cancer survivors could benefit tremendously from a coordinated public health effort to support them. Survivors face numerous physical, psychological, social, spiritual, and financial issues throughout their diagnosis and treatment and for the remaining years of their lives. Many of these issues could be successfully addressed through public health initiatives, both by the prevention of secondary diseases or recurrence of cancer and by improving quality of life for each survivor. A public health effort to address cancer survivorship supports the Healthy People 2010 goal to increase the proportion of cancer survivors who are living 5 years or longer after diagnosis to 70% (USDHHS, 2000). Further, the financial burden of cancer treatment is estimated to be at least $41 billion annually (NCI, 2003b), and this dollar amount does not reflect the burden of cancer on the survivor in every other realm of life. Given this information, it is in the country's best interest to more effectively and systematically provide public health services to cancer survivors.

The Plan

A National Action Plan for Cancer Survivorship: Advancing Public Health Strategies was developed through a partnership between the Centers for Disease Control and Prevention (CDC) and the Lance Armstrong Foundation (LAF) to identify and prioritize cancer survivorship needs that will advance cancer survivorship public health efforts. Specific objectives of the National Action Plan include the following:

- Achieve the cancer survivorship-related objectives in Healthy People 2010 that include benchmarks for success in measuring improvements for addressing ongoing survivor needs.
- Increase awareness among the general public, policy makers, survivors, providers, and others of cancer survivorship and its impact.
- Establish a solid base of applied research and scientific knowledge on the ongoing physical, psychological, social, spiritual, and economic issues facing cancer survivors.
- Identify appropriate mechanisms and resources for ongoing surveillance of people living with, through, and beyond cancer.
- Establish or maintain training for health care professionals to improve delivery of services and increase awareness of issues faced by cancer survivors.
- Implement effective and proven programs and policies to address cancer survivorship more comprehensively.
- Ensure that all cancer survivors have adequate access to high-quality treatment and other post-treatment follow-up services.
- Implement an evaluation methodology that will monitor quality and effectiveness of the outcomes of initiatives.

Once these objectives were identified, CDC and LAF brought together experts in cancer survivorship and public health to create this National Action Plan. Needs and strategies for addressing these needs were discussed within four core public health components:

- Surveillance and applied research
- Communication, education, and training
- Programs, policies, and infrastructure
- Access to quality care and services

This National Action Plan represents these discussions and sets priorities and identifies strategies for national, state, and community-level public health organizations. Given the importance of this health issue—its prevalence, its impact on quality of life, and the resulting costs to survivors and others in their lives—the time for action is now. This National Action Plan should be used to guide the allocation of resources to decrease the burden of cancer for all Americans and improve the overall experience and quality of life of the millions who are living with, through, and beyond cancer.

Carlos, Cancer Survivor

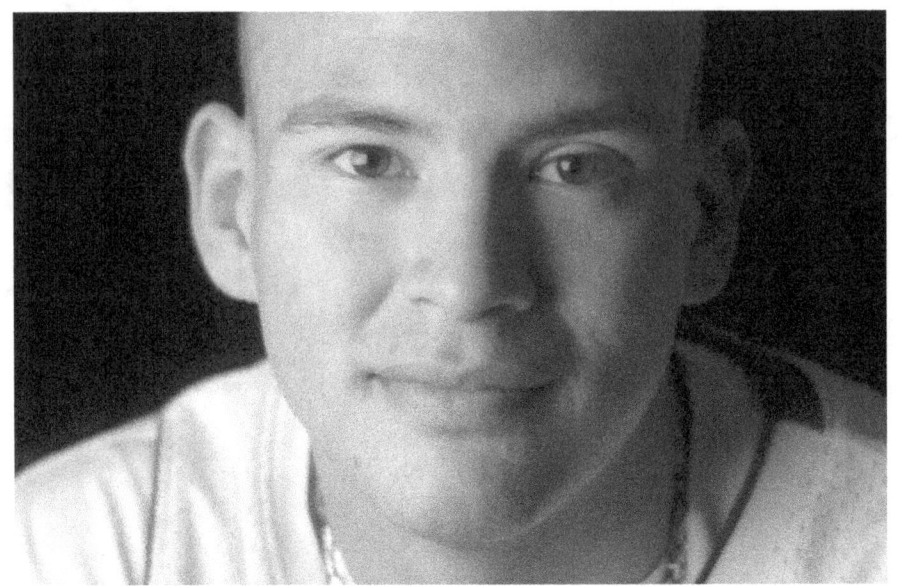

"Survivorship means being given a second chance at life."

I. BACKGROUND

The number of people affected by cancer, both individuals diagnosed with the disease and their families and friends, is staggering. Although all Americans are at **risk** of a cancer diagnosis in their lifetimes, there have been remarkable reductions in deaths associated with cancer. These reductions in deaths are largely due to the implementation of prevention and early detection efforts for certain cancers, increased screening of the general population and those at highest risk for developing these diseases, and advances in research and clinical care. As of January 2000, there were approximately 9.6 million persons living following a cancer diagnosis in the United States (NCI, 2003a) not including family members, friends, and caregivers. This number is expected to increase steadily over the coming years.

A National Action Plan for Cancer Survivorship: Advancing Public Health Strategies was developed through a partnership between the Centers for Disease Control and Prevention (CDC) and the Lance Armstrong Foundation (LAF). Through this partnership and with input from a variety of experts and advocates in public health and cancer survivorship, this National Action Plan charts a course for how the public health community can more effectively and comprehensively address cancer survivorship, including the following:

- Preventing secondary cancers and recurrence of cancer whenever possible.
- Promoting appropriate management following diagnosis and/or treatment to ensure the maximum number of years of healthy life for cancer survivors.
- Minimizing preventable pain, disability, and psychosocial distress for those living with, through, and beyond cancer.
- Supporting cancer survivors in accessing the resources and the family, peer, and community support they need to cope with their disease.

The goal of this National Action Plan is to advance public health efforts regarding cancer survivorship to actively address the needs of this growing population.

The following section describes elements important to understanding the issues cancer survivors face. Throughout this National Action Plan, the term **"cancer survivors"** refers to those people who have been diagnosed with cancer and the people in their lives who are affected by their diagnosis, including family members, friends, and caregivers.

A. The Cancer Burden

Everyone is potentially at risk for developing some form of **cancer**. The American Cancer Society (ACS) predicts that as many as 1.3 million new cancer cases will be diagnosed in 2003 (ACS, 2003). Age is a primary **risk factor** for most cancers, with about 77% of all cancers diagnosed among individuals aged 55 or older. Cancer **incidence** varies by race and ethnicity, with some groups being more likely to be diagnosed with certain types of cancers than others. Cancer is the second leading cause of death in the United States, causing 1 of every 4 deaths each year (ACS, 2004). If current trends continue, one-third of Americans will be diagnosed with cancer in their lifetimes (NCI, 2003a). There is a great deal of misunderstanding about cancer, the effects it can have on those diagnosed with it, and the importance of addressing the ongoing needs of survivors as progress is made in finding treatments and prolonging life after diagnosis.

How many people are expected to survive cancer?
As previously noted, there were approximately 9.6 million persons living following a cancer diagnosis in the United States as of January 2000 (NCI, 2003a) not including family members, friends, and caregivers. Survival rates from cancer depend a great deal on the site where the initial growth began (e.g., breast, colon) and the stage of progression at which the cancer was diagnosed (i.e., whether the growth has **metastasized**). The implementation of prevention (tobacco control and skin protective behavior) and early detection efforts for four cancer types (breast, cervical, colorectal, and prostate), which has increased screening of the general population and those at highest risk for developing these diseases, and advances in research and clinical care have led to remarkable reductions in cancer-related mortality.

Despite the optimistic outlook for most individuals diagnosed with cancer today, a closer examination of the literature and of statistical trends indicates that the benefits of current knowledge about state-of-the-art cancer care are not shared equally by all members of our society (Aziz & Rowland, 2003). When survival rates are broken down by race/ethnicity, it is clear that significant differences exist across racial/ethnic minority and medically underserved populations with respect to the risk of developing and dying from cancer. For all cancer sites combined, African Americans are more likely to develop and die from cancer than persons of any other racial or ethnic group. They are also at greater risk of dying of the four most common types of cancer (lung, breast, colon, and prostate cancer) than any other minority group (ACS, 2004).

B. Redefining Cancer Survivorship

When cancer was considered incurable, the term "survivor" was used to describe family members who survived the loss of a loved one to cancer (Leigh, 1996). As knowledge and success in understanding cancer increased, physicians began to use a 5-year time frame to define survivorship. If cancer did not recur in the 5 years following either diagnosis or treatment, patients were considered to have become "survivors" (Leigh, 1996).

As a result of strong advocacy efforts and coordination led by such organizations as the National Coalition for Cancer Survivorship (NCCS), the term "cancer survivor" has been redefined. The term is now commonly used to describe an individual from the time of diagnosis through the remaining years of life (NCCS, 2003; Leigh, 1996). The National Cancer Institute (NCI) has also expanded this definition to include caregivers and family members within its rubric (Aziz, 2002). This definition—cancer survivor as the person diagnosed with cancer, as well as family members, friends, and caregivers—is the one used in this National Action Plan. The next sections provide an overview of cancer survivorship and describe the issues many survivors face every day.

What are the stages of cancer survivorship?

In "Seasons of Survival: Reflections of a Physician with Cancer," Mullan (1985) was the first to discuss the experience of cancer in terms of a progression of events or stages. He proposed a model of survival that includes three stages: "acute," "extended," and " permanent." The **acute stage** begins with diagnosis and spans the time of further diagnostic and treatment efforts. Mullan describes fear, anxiety, and pain resulting from both illness and treatment as "important and constant elements of this phase." This stage is defined not only by the experience of the person diagnosed with cancer but also by those of the family members who are affected by the diagnosis.

The **extended stage** of survival begins when the survivor goes into remission or has completed treatment. Psychologically, this stage is a time of watchful waiting, with the individual wondering if symptoms may be signs of recurrence or just a part of everyday life. Cancer could return at the same site or in a new location. When treatment is complete, diminished contact with the health care team can also cause great anxiety. Physically, it is a period of continued limitation resulting from having had both illness and treatment. During this stage, survivors may be learning to live with chronic side effects and accompanying anxieties.

The **permanent stage** is defined as a time when the "activity of the disease or likelihood of its return is sufficiently small that the cancer can now be considered permanently arrested" (Mullan, 1985, p. 272). Mullan acknowledges, however, that this stage is more complex than simply the status of disease: a person in this stage may still face social and economic challenges, such as problems with employment and insurance, psychological challenges, the fear of recurrence, and secondary effects from previous cancer treatment.

End-of-life issues can occur during any of the three stages. **End-of-life care** affirms life and regards dying as a normal process, neither hastening nor postponing death while providing relief from distress and integrating psychological and spiritual aspects of survivor care. The goal of end-of-life care is to achieve the best possible quality of life for cancer survivors by controlling pain and other symptoms and addressing psychological and spiritual needs.

Following the work of Mullan (1985) and Leigh (1996), LAF defines the experience of cancer survivorship as living "with," "through," and "beyond" cancer. **Living "with" cancer** refers to the experience of receiving a cancer diagnosis and any treatment that may follow, **living "through" cancer** refers to the extended stage following treatment, and **living "beyond" cancer** refers to post-treatment and long-term survivorship. Although this definition is designed to signify the experience of survivorship as a progression, this process is unique for each patient, and movement from one phase to the next may not be clearly delineated.

C. Issues for Cancer Survivors

How does cancer affect individuals?
Diagnosis of cancer is a threat to a person's physical, psychological, social, spiritual, and economic well-being. During its various stages, cancer can deprive persons diagnosed with it of their independence and can disrupt the lives of family members and other caregivers.

Physical symptoms of cancer can be both acute and chronic and can occur during and after treatment. Physical symptoms may include pain, fatigue, nausea, hair loss, and others, depending on the cancer site and the types of treatments a patient receives. The symptoms experienced by some people with cancer can be debilitating and may result in bed rest. Adequate **palliative care** to provide **pain and symptom management** through every stage of cancer and its treatment is a major concern for survivors. The late or long-term physical effects of cancer itself and/or its treatment can include decreased sexual functioning, loss of fertility, persistent edema, fatigue, chronic pain, and major disabilities. These effects can be devastating, resulting in a loss of mobility (e.g., loss of leg, spinal injury) and changes in bodily functions (e.g., colostomy, laryngectomy) and appearance (e.g., disfiguring surgery, amputation). Major physical issues that affect long-term survival include recurrence of the original disease, development of secondary cancers, premature aging, and organ/systems failure.

Psychological issues associated with cancer diagnosis and treatment includes fear, stress, depression, anger, and anxiety. However, the effects of cancer on an individual are not always negative. Cancer can also provide opportunities for people to find renewed meaning in their lives, build stronger connections with loved ones, and foster a commitment to "give back" to others who go through similar experiences. After cancer diagnosis and/or treatment, survivors can continue to live active, vital lives—but they may live with the uncertainty and the fear that cancer might return. People with cancer may also experience difficulties in coping with pain and disability caused by either their disease or the treatment they are undergoing. Emotional impacts on survivors can include feelings of helplessness, lack of self-control, changes to self-esteem and self-image for the survivor, and added stress and anxiety for their caregivers (NCI, 2002).

Social well-being can be affected by cancer diagnosis and treatment through the physical and psychological impacts discussed above. The physical difficulties of pain and disability may result in a decreased sense of social well-being by limiting the time survivors are able to spend with important people in their lives. Survivors also often experience increased difficulties in school or on the job, in terms of their ability to interact with friends and coworkers, because of the impact diagnosis and treatment can have on their self-image (NCI, 2003b).

Spirituality can take many different forms in the lives of cancer survivors; it can come from organized religion or from personal beliefs and faith. Some survivors struggle with spirituality as part of their cancer experience and say that their faith has been tested. Others gain support from their faith and allow it to guide them through their experience (NCI, 2002). Surviving cancer is a complicated journey that takes its toll on the spirit as well as the body. Some survivors wrestle with "why me" questions about having a cancer diagnosis or experience survivors' guilt because they lived through their diagnosis while others have died. Spiritually, survivors may deal with unresolved grief, reevaluate their lives, reprioritize their goals and ambitions, and redefine "normal" for themselves. Cancer survivors are often looking for guidance and strength to help them through the spiritual journey. In many cases, survivors' spirituality helps them to understand the meaning of their cancer experience and embrace life with a renewed vigor and sense of purpose. Survivors often gain strength through their faith; this strength allows survivors and their loved ones to answer tough questions and to face each day with love and confidence (NCI, 2002).

Economic costs incurred by survivors and their families are another important consideration. Cost implications of cancer include inability to access quality care, financial burdens resulting from health care costs, and income loss resulting from work limitations. Often, survivors have to cope with losing a job because of their employers' preconceived notions about the impact cancer will have on their work capabilities. With job changes, survivors may be unable to qualify for health insurance and often find it difficult to obtain life insurance after diagnosis. Family members of cancer patients may experience significant financial burdens while serving in the role of caretaker, especially during the end-of-life phase. Similarities or differences in the survivorship experience among different racial or ethnic groups or among medically underserved people are virtually unexplored.

What are the common myths about cancer and
cancer survivorship?

There are many myths and misunderstandings about cancer and the
effects it can have on survivors. The following table summarizes some
selected myths and the facts to counteract these misconceptions.

Common Myth	Facts to Counter Myth
Cancer is a disease that only affects older people.	Although approximately 77% of all cancer cases are diagnosed at age 55 or older, everyone is at risk of developing some form of cancer (ACS, 2003).
Cancer only affects the person diagnosed with the disease.	For many years, the focus of cancer diagnosis and treatment was on the person diagnosed with the disease. However, recent advances in our understanding of survivorship have led to the expanded definition of "survivor" to include others touched by this disease, such as families, friends, and caregivers.
Cancer is the same for everyone.	Because cancer can occur anywhere within the body, survivors can experience different symptoms depending on the site of their diagnosis. Depending on the site of the initial cancer growth and the stage at diagnosis, the available treatments and resources will vary greatly, such that more services and resources are available to survivors of certain cancers (e.g., breast or leukemia) than for other rarer forms of cancer (e.g., myeloma or laryngeal).
The need for care of survivors ends once treatment is complete.	Cancer can be a **chronic disease** that often has long-term effects on a survivor's life. Although many cancers can now be cured or the growth greatly slowed, the impacts of diagnosis will remain with a survivor for years. Because more survivors are living longer, especially those diagnosed with cancer as a child or young adult, there is a need to address long-term issues of survivorship. These can include ongoing physical, psychological, and other types of issues (see Section I.C.)
Diagnosis of cancer means certain death.	The risk of dying of cancer following diagnosis has steadily decreased over the past several decades. Fewer than half the people diagnosed with cancer today will die of the disease; in fact, some are completely cured, and many more survive for years because of early diagnosis or treatments that control many types of cancer (ACS, 2004).

Although many dedicated individuals and organizations have contributed to reductions in the number of cancer diagnoses and an increase in the likelihood of survival following diagnosis, much remains to be done. An ever-growing population of cancer survivors is in need of medical care, public health services, and support. All of these factors need to be taken into account when assessing the experience of cancer survivorship.

D. Public Health and Cancer Survivorship

A primary purpose of this National Action Plan is to identify areas within the realm of **public health** that can be mobilized to address the needs of cancer survivors. Although the role of biomedical research is to increase our understanding of the causes and physical effects of cancer, responsibility for applying knowledge about potential interventions that can be implemented to eradicate disease and/or improve the quality of life rests within both the medical care and public health communities. Because cancer survivorship imposes a tremendous individual and societal burden and proven interventions are available to address survivor needs, a coordinated public health effort is warranted. The focus of that effort should be broad and encompass entire population groups, in contrast with the medical model, which generally focuses on individual patients. The following provides an overview of public health and existing infrastructure that can be used to initiate efforts for cancer survivors.

What is public health?

Public health practice is the science and art of preventing disease, prolonging life, and promoting health and well-being (Winslow, 1923). More recently, the Institute of Medicine (IOM) (1998) has defined the mission of public health as assuring conditions in which people can be healthy. Public health's mission is achieved through the application of health promotion and disease prevention technologies and interventions designed to improve and enhance quality of life (PHFSC, 1994). Health promotion and disease prevention technologies encompass a broad array of functions and expertise, including the 3 core public health functions and 10 essential public health services presented in the following table.

Three Core Public Health Functions
• Assess and monitor the health of communities and populations at risk to identify health problems and priorities.
• Formulate public policies, in collaboration with community and government leaders, designed to solve identified local and national health problems and priorities.
• Assure that all populations have access to appropriate and cost-effective care, including health promotion and disease prevention services, and evaluation of the effectiveness of that care.

Ten Essential Public Health Services
• Monitor health status to identify community health problems.
• Diagnose and investigate health problems and health hazards in the community.
• Inform, educate, and empower people about health issues.
• Mobilize community partnerships to identify and solve health problems.
• Develop policies and plans that support individual and community health efforts.
• Enforce laws and regulations that protect health and ensure safety.
• Link people to needed personal health services and assure the provision of health care when otherwise unavailable.
• Assure a competent public health and personal health care workforce.
• Evaluate effectiveness, accessibility, and quality of personal and population-based health services.
• Research for new insights and innovative solutions to health problems.

Source: Public Health Functions Steering Committee (PHFSC), 1994.

What is the relevant public health infrastructure for addressing cancer survivorship?

Two agencies within the U.S. Department of Health and Human Services—the National Institutes of Health (NIH) and CDC—have been established to conduct research and implement public health strategies to address cancer. Within NIH, NCI works to reduce the burden of cancer **morbidity** and mortality among Americans. NCI's goal is to stimulate and support scientific discovery and its application to achieve a future when all cancers are uncommon and easily treated. Through basic and clinical biomedical research and training, NCI conducts and supports research programs to understand the causes of cancer; prevent, detect, diagnose, treat, and control cancer; and disseminate information to the practitioner, patient, and public (NIH, 2003). NCI works to "enhance the quality and length of survival of all persons diagnosed with cancer and to minimize or

stabilize adverse effects experienced during cancer survivorship"
(NIH, 2003). Through its conduct and support of research, NCI
works to effectively address all issues facing cancer survivors (see
Section I.C.).

Within the CDC, the National Center for Chronic Disease
Prevention and Health Promotion works to prevent cancer and to
increase early detection of cancer. CDC works with partners in the
government, private, and nonprofit sectors to develop, implement,
and promote effective cancer early detection, prevention, and
control practices nationwide (CDC, 2003a). Within the CDC, the
National Comprehensive Cancer Control (CCC) Program
provides a mechanism for addressing cancer survivorship within the
realm of public health.

Background on the CDC's Comprehensive Cancer Control Program

CDC began implementing the CCC Program through state health
departments and other entities in the mid-1990s and defines this
Program as "an integrated and coordinated approach to reducing
cancer incidence, morbidity, and mortality through prevention,
early detection, treatment, rehabilitation, and palliation" (CDC,
2002, p. 1). This strategy aims to engage and build a coordinated
public health response and provide a way to assess and then address
the cancer burden within a state, territory, or tribal organization.
Not only do state-level CCC Programs build on the achievements of
cancer programs, they enhance the infrastructure created for them—
many of which focus on individual cancer sites or risk factors.
Partnerships between public and private **stakeholders** whose
common mission is to reduce the overall burden of cancer provide
the foundation for these statewide programs:

**"These stakeholders review epidemiologic data and research evidence
(including program evaluation data) and then jointly set priorities for
action. The partnership then mobilizes support for implementing these
priorities and puts in place a systematic plan to institutionalize the
comprehensive approach as a means to coordinate activities, monitor
progress over time, and reassess priorities periodically in light of emerging
developments in cancer and related fields" (CDC, 2002, p. 2).**

Public health agencies are using this support to establish broad-
based cancer coalitions, assess the burden of cancer, determine
priorities for cancer prevention and control, and develop and

implement comprehensive plans, most of which include addressing the needs of cancer survivors.

E. Summary

A National Action Plan for Cancer Survivorship: Advancing Public Health Strategies was developed to identify and prioritize cancer survivorship needs and strategies within the context of public health that will ultimately improve the overall experience and quality of life of the millions of Americans who are living with, through, and beyond cancer. It can be used by state agencies, organizations, and individuals in selecting and developing activities to comprehensively address cancer survivorship. The primary outcomes of this National Action Plan are to increase awareness among the general public, policy makers, researchers, advocates, survivors, and others of the role public health can play in advancing cancer survivorship issues and to stimulate organizations to take action to meet the identified needs in surveillance and applied research; communication, education, and training; programs, policies, and infrastructure; and access to quality care and services.

Theodore, Cancer Survivor

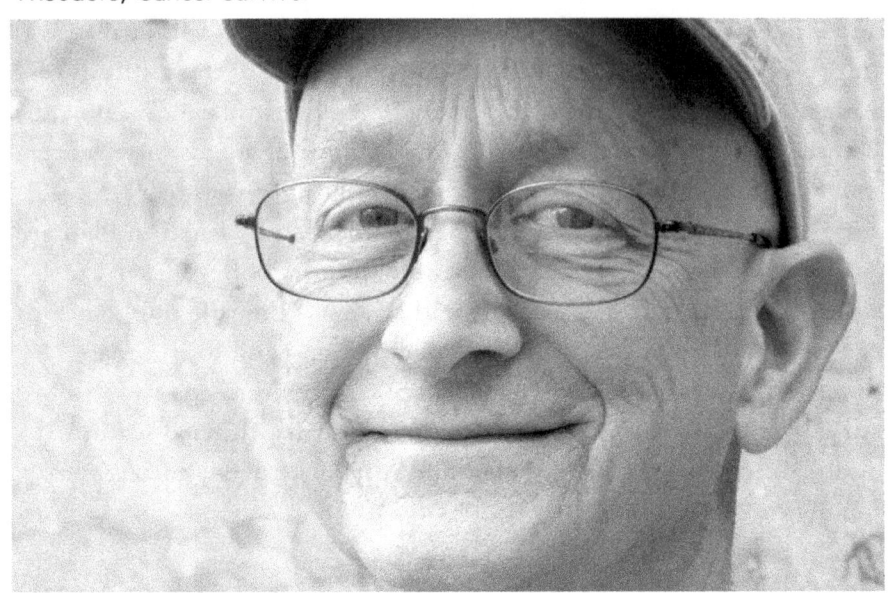

"Survivorship means more time and responsibility — time for family, friends, work and life."

II. STRATEGIC FRAMEWORK

CDC and LAF collaborated in 2002 to comprehensively address cancer survivorship within the realm of public health. Through a series of subsequent meetings among key partners (Appendix A), areas within public health that could be enhanced to address cancer survivorship were identified.

To expand these efforts to additional partners, including numerous organizations, advocates, survivors, and researchers, the CDC and the LAF conducted a workshop in June 2003 entitled Building Partnerships to Advance Cancer Survivorship and Public Health. This 2-day workshop brought together nearly 100 experts from multiple disciplines to discuss how public health can be mobilized to address cancer survivorship in the identified public health areas. Using the core public health functions and services as a guide (see Section I.D.), participants were led through a process to identify priority needs in the following four identified topic areas within the realm of public health:

- Surveillance and applied research
- Communication, education, and training
- Programs, policies, and infrastructure
- Access to quality care and services

The culmination of these efforts is *A National Action Plan for Cancer Survivorship: Advancing Public Health Strategies*. This National Action Plan provides a vision and a framework for addressing the problems faced by cancer survivors in our nation. It further proposes strategic initiatives that would constitute a coordinated, responsible approach within the entire public health structure, including at the national, state, and community levels. This National Action Plan is groundbreaking in that it outlines a comprehensive, systematic public health approach to acknowledging and addressing cancer survivorship.

A. Purpose

The goal of this National Action Plan is to identify and prioritize cancer survivorship needs and identify strategies within public health to address those needs that will ultimately lead to improved quality of life for the millions of Americans who are living with, through, and beyond cancer. A first step in addressing these needs is to develop strong partnerships with health professionals, researchers, survivors, advocates, and other key stakeholders. These partnerships will serve to identify and prioritize the steps necessary to integrate cancer survivorship issues into the public health domain. Outcomes of the National Action Plan's development include the following:

- Laying the foundation for public health activities in cancer survivorship.
- Identifying, discussing, and prioritizing strategies to expand and enhance the role of public health agencies and practitioners in cancer survivorship.
- Facilitating the development and enhancement of collaborations and partnerships that will assist with the expansion of public health's role in cancer survivorship.

B. Overarching Goals and Objectives

The overarching goal of this National Action Plan is to establish a coordinated national effort for addressing cancer survivorship within the realm of public health. Specific objectives include the following:

- Achieve the cancer survivorship-related objectives in **Healthy People 2010** (Appendix B) that include benchmarks for success in measuring improvements for addressing ongoing survivor needs.
- Increase awareness among the general public, policy makers, survivors, and others of cancer survivorship and its impact.
- Establish a solid base of applied research and scientific knowledge on the ongoing physical, psychological, social, spiritual, and economic issues facing cancer survivors.
- Identify appropriate mechanisms and resources for ongoing surveillance of people living with, through, and beyond cancer.
- Establish or maintain training for health care professionals to improve delivery of services and increase awareness of issues faced by cancer survivors.
- Implement effective and proven programs and policies to address cancer survivorship more comprehensively.
- Ensure that all cancer survivors have adequate access to high-quality treatment and other post-treatment follow-up services.
- Implement an evaluation methodology that will monitor quality and effectiveness of the outcomes of this initiative.

C. Guidelines for the National Action Plan

Addressing and achieving the National Action Plan's goals and objectives require a multifaceted approach that is both ambitious and feasible. The National Action Plan consists of prioritized needs and strategies in four major areas of public health work, which are defined below: surveillance and applied research; communication, education, and training; programs, policies, and infrastructure; and access to quality care and services.

C.1 Surveillance and Applied Research

Surveillance and applied research are the scientific tools of public health and can be used to establish a solid, systematic knowledge base in cancer survivorship.

Surveillance

Cancer surveillance is the systematic collection, analysis, and use of cancer data. Information obtained through surveillance measures is critical for directing effective cancer prevention and control programs (CDC, 2001). Primary surveillance measures include cancer registries and several national and regional/state surveys. Cancer registries (National Program of Cancer Registries [NPCR]; Surveillance, Epidemiology, and End Results [SEER] Program) implement and maintain information systems designed to collect and manage data on each newly diagnosed case of cancer. National surveys, such as the National Health Interview Survey (NHIS) and the Behavioral Risk Factor Surveillance System (BRFSS), provide information on health attitudes, beliefs, and behaviors that could be used to help understand issues related to all stages of cancer survivorship.

Applied Research

Cancer survivorship research in a public health context would focus efforts on applying our knowledge of cancer and issues survivors face to the development of appropriate interventions. Understanding specific structural, policy, or behavioral barriers to desired outcomes and evaluating programmatic efforts are other examples of applied research. Applied research investigates the extent to which these efforts effectively address survivor needs and provides findings that can guide further development of initiatives.

C.2 Communication, Education, and Training

Communication, education, and training include efforts to communicate with the general public and policy and decision makers, educate survivors and their families, and train **health care providers**

to meet informational needs of all those affected by cancer survivorship.

Communication with the Public
___

Communication with the general public and policy or decision makers about the issues surrounding cancer survivorship aims to create a societal understanding and acceptance of the growing population of cancer survivors and the issues they face.

Survivor Education
___

Education of cancer survivors includes provision of information tailored to the particular stage of survivorship. Such educational interventions may be most appropriate during the first 5 years after diagnosis as this is the time when many of the challenges associated with the adjustment to survivorship occur (Mullan, 1984).

Provider Training
___

Health care provider training aims to ensure that providers are aware of the medical and other special needs of cancer survivors so they can offer the spectrum of services available to enhance quality of life throughout survivorship and refer survivors to these services as appropriate.

C.3 Programs, Policies, and Infrastructure
Programs, policies, and infrastructure are the means by which change can be made in public health.

Programs
___

Programs are the actual implementation of specific interventions at the national, state, and community levels to address a public health problem (NAAP, 1999). Medical, psychosocial, legal, and financial issues could be addressed by programs that are comprehensive in scope and encompass care for each stage of cancer survivorship.

Policies
___

Policies include legislation, regulations, ordinances, guidelines, and norms that establish an environment conducive to program implementation and other changes specific to survivorship (NAAP, 1999). These policies may be implemented at the national, state, organizational, and community levels in an effort to advance public health.

Infrastructure

Infrastructure is comprised of the basic resources and facilities in place to address survivorship and includes components of the health care and public health systems, such as state and local health departments, and the services and programs they provide. Effective infrastructure is required to operate and manage effective programs. As our health care system continues to evolve, delivery of quality care becomes more complex. Relationships among the public and private sectors, individual practitioners and managed care organizations, and voluntary health organizations directly influence access to care and provision of clinical and community services (NAAP, 1999).

C.4 Access to Quality Care and Services

Access to quality care and services means ensuring that survivors have access to evidence-based and appropriate treatment and services delivered in a timely and technically competent manner, with good communication, shared decision making between the cancer survivor and health care providers, and cultural sensitivity across the continuum of care and throughout the remainder of life (IOM, 1999). Public health can play a role in identifying and disseminating proven programs in the following areas to groups of cancer survivors.

Access to Quality Treatment

Cancer treatment is complex and differs for each individual based on his or her specific situation and needs. All cancer patients should have timely access to the latest and most effective treatments available. This would include **clinical trials**, if appropriate.

Pain and Symptom Management

An important part of cancer treatment is the management of pain and other symptoms associated with both disease and treatment. The goal of pain and symptom management is to provide relief so that survivors can tolerate the diagnostic and therapeutic procedures needed to treat their cancer and live comfortably throughout each stage of cancer survivorship.

End-of-Life Care

Issues facing survivors and their families during end-of-life are complex and serious. Appropriate end-of-life care affirms life and regards dying as a normal process, neither hastening nor postponing death. The goal of end-of-life care is to achieve the best possible quality of life for cancer survivors. Although many survivors live many years beyond their diagnosis, the needs and desires of those who are in the process of dying must be addressed.

Lindy, Cancer Survivor

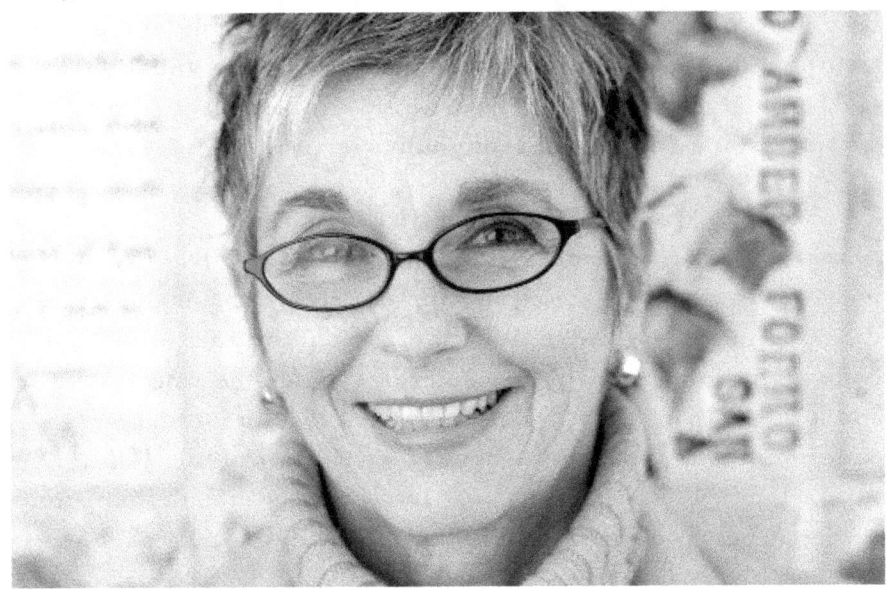

"Survivorship means I get to watch my grandchildren growing up."

III. CROSS-CUTTING NEEDS AND STRATEGIES

Four primary topic areas (see Section II.C.) for advancing cancer survivorship within the realm of public health have been identified:

- Surveillance and applied research
- Communication, education, and training
- Programs, policies, and infrastructure
- Access to quality care and services

Within these topic areas, five specific cross-cutting needs were identified.

1. Develop an infrastructure for a comprehensive database on cancer survivorship.

Increasing the capacity of surveillance systems to capture information on health topics of interest can lead to a better understanding of diseases and the people affected by them. Effective survivorship research is dependent upon the integration and interaction of many information sources that serve as a strong and comprehensive infrastructure for study. A comprehensive database system could provide information on the ongoing health and other issues facing survivors. It could also provide the opportunity to follow survivors for many years after cancer diagnosis in order to better understand the long-term effects of having this disease. Enhancing the existing surveillance and research infrastructure can also ultimately lead to the development and implementation of strategies identified for other topic areas outlined in this National Action Plan. The following strategies focus on the specific data needs for cancer survivorship that have been identified to enhance the existing surveillance systems and applied research initiatives:

- Develop a national Work Group or Task Force composed of diverse organizations, representing private, nonprofit, and governmental agencies, to identify data needs for ongoing follow-up and confidential monitoring of cancer survivorship issues (e.g., treatment course and outcomes, quality-of-life indicators, long-term effects of diagnosis and treatment).
- Assess existing data on cancer survivors to identify gaps in order to determine areas of future research.
- Develop consensus on a set of data items or **indicators** used in the collection and analysis of cancer survivorship data, including data needed for long-term follow-up on survivors.

- Improve coordination among existing databases (e.g., NPCR, BRFSS, SEER), and add data variables or indicators where possible to collect supplementary information on cancer survivors.
- Develop a centralized resource center (i.e., clearinghouse) that includes linkages to all existing data sources and that provides for longitudinal data collection, monitoring, and follow-up.
- Increase the number and types of funding opportunities to enable a broader range of researchers to participate in survivorship surveillance activities.
- Use existing information technology to gather data on cancer diagnosis, treatment, and long-term issues and report the data in a timely manner.
- Provide widespread access to public data sets as quickly as possible to enhance research activities.

2. Develop, test, maintain, and promote patient navigation systems that can facilitate optimum care for cancer survivors. Patient navigation is a tool that can be used to ensure that survivors understand their care and their process of care, and to enhance the delivery of optimum care. In these programs, health professionals and highly trained patient liaison representatives coordinate health care for patients and assist them in navigating the health care system. These navigators can provide information that will help educate the survivor about his or her health needs and concerns, ensure timely delivery of care, connect survivors with appropriate resources that will meet their needs, and provide general oversight to the delivery and payment of services for each survivor. Key strategies for developing and maintaining these programs include the following:

- Establish infrastructure of the patient navigation system, consisting of appropriate existing national organizations, to implement a national program with consistent delivery of services for cancer survivors.
- Promote universal input and buy-in by having patient navigation system co-branded and co-owned by all appropriate organizations.
- Identify existing types of patient navigation systems delivered in a variety of locations or through different mechanisms (e.g., rural, urban, on-line, print, telephone, clinical trials), and determine those that are considered **best practices**.

- Develop a database of existing and tested patient navigator tools/programs and educate survivors and others at the national, state, and community levels on their use.
- Plan, develop, and incorporate patient navigation systems into state comprehensive cancer control plans.
- Develop policies to require insurance coverage of patient navigation services.
- Develop effective patient navigator tools that address issues of disparity (e.g., race, ethnicity, education, geography, income, gender) among survivors.
- Encourage cancer survivors to volunteer their time (**in-kind**) to serve as individual navigators servicing other survivors.

3. Establish and /or disseminate clinical practice guidelines for each stage of cancer survivorship.

Clinical practice guidelines are defined by the IOM as "…systematically developed statements to assist practitioner and patient decisions for specific clinical circumstances" (IOM, 1992). These guidelines summarize the collective research on outcomes pertaining to one disease. When using the guidelines, physicians have to select from among the guideline recommendations those that seem most applicable to each individual's care. In their statement, "Principles of Quality Cancer Care," the Cancer Leadership Council emphasizes that all people with cancer need to have timely access to care that is based on the best available evidence (NCCS, 2003). Treatment options should include access to clinical trials, therapies to manage side effects, and services to help survivors and caregivers cope with emotional and practical concerns. Guidelines have been developed for the treatment of particular cancers, but they are not necessarily comprehensive in the sense of specifying care for survivors at each stage of cancer survivorship (e.g., monitoring survivors after treatment is completed, monitoring long-term health care). Guidelines are also in place to address end-of-life care so that survivors do not suffer from intense pain and discomfort during the final stages of life (IOM, 1997). The following strategies are proposed to systematically move toward quality and timely service provision so that guidelines are available throughout every stage of living with, through, and beyond cancer:

- Charge appropriate groups working on cancer survivorship issues (e.g., National Comprehensive Cancer Network, American Society of Clinical Oncology, NCCS) to develop clinical practice guidelines specific to each stage of cancer survivorship.

- Establish a centralized location for housing these guidelines (e.g., National Guidelines Clearinghouse, Cancer Information Service [CIS]).
- Develop both consumer and health care provider versions of each clinical practice guideline and disseminate through multiple channels and organizations.
- Require that programs funded by public health organizations include implementation of clinical practice guidelines (e.g., state cancer plans, CCC Programs).
- Ensure accessibility of services named in each clinical practice guideline.
- Conduct ongoing evaluation of guidelines and use results to assess utilization. Modify guidelines as needed.
- Provide training to cancer and non-cancer health professionals about guidelines to maximize workforce development.
- Ensure quality workforce by requiring ongoing training on such topics as cultural sensitivity and palliative care.
- Assess gaps in the health care workforce and develop strategies to recruit and retain quality service providers.

4. Develop and disseminate public education programs that empower cancer survivors to make informed decisions.

No one medical answer is right for everyone. Cancer survivors are faced with extremely difficult medical decisions at each stage of living with, through, and beyond cancer. In making difficult medical decisions, survivors need to thoroughly understand their options for care and why it is in their best interest to participate fully in the decision-making process. The informed decision-making process also enables physicians to more fully understand the attitudes and values of their patients, especially those with diverse cultural backgrounds. A growing body of research shows that when patients are well-informed and play a significant role in deciding how they are going to manage their health, the results are more positive. Informed patients feel better about the outcomes of the decision-making process and are therefore more likely to follow their providers' recommendations (Mulley, 1995). Key strategies for addressing this need include the following:

- Form a national Task Force to develop programs addressing public education among survivors, and create a multifaceted strategic plan around this issue.

- Identify existing resources available to survivors to facilitate informed decision making and advocacy skills, and develop programs or materials where information is lacking.
- Charge the national Task Force with implementing marketing strategies and a multimedia campaign to effectively educate survivors about issues and available education programs, using numerous modes for communication (e.g., Internet, print media).
- Disseminate and encourage implementation of best practices for enhancing informed decision making through a variety of venues (e.g., health care providers, advocacy groups, government agencies, legislators).

5. Conduct ongoing evaluation of all activities to determine their impacts and outcomes and ensure continuous quality improvement of services.

Evaluation planning and implementation are important processes in program development. The ultimate goals of these processes are to assess program implementation and outcomes, to increase program efficiency and impact over time, and to demonstrate accountability (CDC, 2001). According to CDC's "Framework for Program Evaluation in Public Health" (1999), program evaluation is an essential organizational practice in public health. The Framework proposes that evaluation is necessary to use science as a basis for decision making and public health action, expand the quest for social equity through public health action, perform effectively as a service agency, make efforts outcome-oriented, and be accountable (CDC, 1999). For evaluation to be effectively implemented, quality indicators need to be developed for programs and services so that progress toward articulated goals can be measured. These evaluation efforts should be continuous so that improvements can be made during all phases of program implementation. The following strategies could be used to comprehensively include evaluation and quality improvement in addressing all needs:

- Identify evaluation measures for each type of program or strategy implemented from the National Action Plan.
- Conduct theoretically-based and scientifically-grounded studies to assess implementation.
- Disseminate evidence-based program evaluation findings through public health organizations and other venues in order to maximize use of information.

Section III Summary:
Cross-Cutting Needs for Cancer Survivors

1. Develop an infrastructure for a comprehensive database on cancer survivorship.

2. Develop, test, maintain, and promote patient navigation systems that can facilitate optimum care for cancer survivors.

3. Establish and/or disseminate clinical practice guidelines for each stage of cancer survivorship.

4. Develop and disseminate public education programs that empower cancer survivors to make informed decisions.

5. Conduct ongoing evaluation of all activities to determine their impacts and outcomes and ensure continuous quality improvement of services.

Jan, Breast Cancer Survivor

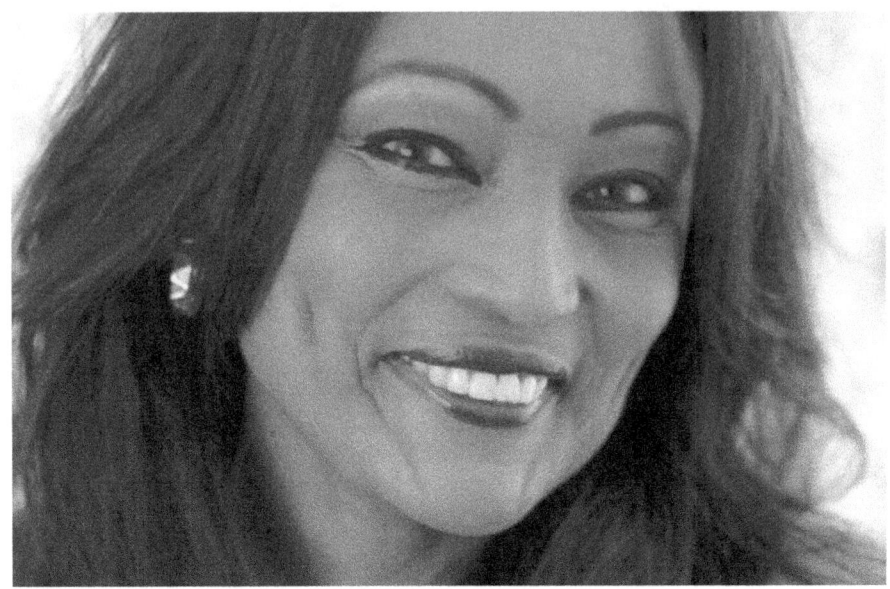

"Survivorship is the ultimate understanding of one's purpose in life."

IV. SURVEILLANCE AND APPLIED RESEARCH

A. Goals

Surveillance and applied research are integral elements of any public health initiative. Surveillance provides data items or indicators on diseases and populations affected by them in order to understand what is associated with diagnosis, health care outcomes, and numerous other variables. Applied research uses these data to better understand how initiatives can be designed to more effectively address and meet the needs of groups of people. For cancer survivorship, goals for this topic area include the following:

- Enhance the existing infrastructure to create a comprehensive surveillance system that can be used to understand the range of health issues that cancer survivors face and any differences between survivor groups based on demographic and medical variables.
- Thoroughly understand the factors associated with susceptibility to problems during each stage of cancer survivorship.
- Translate the research on cancer survivorship into practice by developing, implementing, and evaluating effective health intervention strategies.

Surveillance and applied research are the scientific tools of public health and are defined here and in Section II.C. as follows:

Surveillance

Cancer surveillance is the systematic collection, analysis, and use of cancer data. Information obtained through surveillance measures is critical for directing effective cancer prevention and control programs (CDC, 2001). Primary surveillance measures include cancer registries and several national and regional/state surveys. Cancer registries (NPCR, SEER) implement and maintain information systems designed to collect and manage data on each newly diagnosed case of cancer. National surveys, such as the NHIS and BRFSS, provide information on health attitudes, beliefs, and behaviors that could be used to help understand issues related to all stages of cancer survivorship.

Applied Research

Cancer survivorship research in a public health context would focus efforts on applying our knowledge of cancer and issues survivors face to the development of appropriate interventions. Understanding specific structural, policy, or behavioral barriers to desired outcomes and evaluating programmatic efforts are other examples of applied research. Applied research investigates the extent to which these efforts effectively address survivor needs and provides findings that can guide further development of initiatives.

Prioritized needs for these components and suggested strategies for addressing them are presented in the following section.

B. Prioritized Needs and Suggested Strategies

1. Enhance the existing surveillance and applied research infrastructure.

Increasing the capacity of surveillance systems to capture information on health topics of interest can lead to a better understanding of diseases and the people affected by them. Effective survivorship research is dependent upon the integration and interaction of many information sources that serve as a strong and comprehensive infrastructure for study. A surveillance system that provides data on the long-term effects of cancer is critical to advancing survivorship. This need is described in detail in Section III of this *National Action Plan*.

2. Identify factors associated with ongoing health concerns of cancer survivors.

As described in Section I, only within the past two decades have research and knowledge demonstrated that cancer is a disease a person can survive for many years after treatment. With their successful survival from cancer diagnosis and treatment, survivors are often faced with ongoing health concerns, such as heart problems, major disabilities, **lymphedema**, infertility, and others (NCI, 2002). Although there is understanding of the types of health problems cancer diagnosis and treatment may cause immediately, less is known about the long-term effects and how different people are affected by the services they receive. Some people may be prone to certain types of complications or long-term difficulties, but little is known that can help prevent or educate survivors on avoiding these problems. The extent to which diagnosis and treatment of cancer may impact the chances that a survivor will later develop other, secondary diseases is also unknown. Assessments of the potential for these problems can help guide delivery of health services to prevent or encourage early detection of other cancers and health complications (e.g., diabetes, heart disease) and thereby improve the quality of life for survivors. In addition, knowing the characteristics of survivors who are more prone to develop ongoing complications can help researchers, policy and decision makers, program managers, and others to direct the development and implementation of survivorship services and programs that will address specific needs. Strategies to address this need include the following:

- Initiate research studies to identify characteristics associated with certain types of cancer and/or secondary health concerns.
- Identify modifiable behaviors (e.g., limited physical activity, poor eating habits) that can be targeted with interventions to reduce the likelihood of additional health problems.
- Once more is known about which characteristics render survivors susceptible to health problems (e.g., different age groups), develop **primary prevention** education programs to inform survivors about their susceptibility and any behavioral changes they can make to reduce their risk.

3. Determine programs and services that best address the needs of cancer survivors.

Once more is understood about the health concerns survivors may face—particularly those that occur long after treatment ends—and the groups of survivors most susceptible to them, programs and services can be delivered to maximize the chances of optimum health among survivors during each stage of living with, through, and beyond cancer. These programs and services can include providing adequate screening for cancer recurrence (e.g., more frequent follow-up screening exams for those diagnosed with screen-detectable cancers than is recommended for the general population), follow-up surveillance of health concerns (e.g., frequent testing for heart problems among survivors of childhood cancers [IOM, 2003]), psychological and/or support group services, planning for possible infertility, and additional services that can be made strategically available to those most susceptible to recurring problems. More needs to be understood about the types of programs and services to provide survivors and the point in time at which these interventions would have the greatest positive impact. Importantly, the characteristics of those survivors most likely to benefit from delivery of developed services need to be identified. Strategies to meet this need include the following:

- Gain a better understanding of how cancer survivors interact with the health care system by conducting national surveys (e.g., NHIS, BRFSS) to delineate the services delivered, usage pattern, and any problems in these areas.

- Enhance collaborative efforts among academic researchers and state health departments to develop research projects to increase the body of knowledge about the care and services that can be provided to survivors to reduce susceptibility to additional health problems.
- Identify, evaluate, and disseminate findings of the most effective models of survivorship care.
- Incorporate lessons learned from this body of knowledge into state comprehensive cancer control plans.

4. Conduct research on preventive interventions to evaluate their impact on issues related to cancer survivorship.

Preventive interventions are those programs, activities, and services that identify areas of behavior that can be changed to reduce cancer recurrence and promote healthy lifestyles. The scope of preventive interventions includes, but is not limited to, reducing tobacco and alcohol use and sun exposure; improving nutrition, mental health, and early detection or follow-up, such as survivor self-advocacy; and increasing physical activity. This work is important not only for preventing other cancers and diseases but also for reducing cancer recurrence. Specific strategies for conducting this research include the following:

- Develop an inventory of existing preventive interventions.
- Evaluate programs in different public health settings to determine the effectiveness of a particular intervention and establish best practices for cancer survivors.
- Identify gaps in existing interventions through evaluation research.
- Develop interventions that address people at highest risk for developing other cancers and/or secondary health conditions.
- Conduct cost-effectiveness research of selected interventions.
- Customize communication to specific cancer survivor populations, with a specific focus on underserved communities, to increase awareness of available interventions and resources.

5. Translate applied research into practice.

Translating scientific research into practice is a crucial step in increasing the quality of life of cancer survivors. Research findings should be utilized to develop and implement programs and services that reduce negative health effects and promote long-term health benefits. In turn, these programs will benefit cancer survivors by enhancing the health care services that they receive. The following strategies would begin to address this need:

- Incorporate cancer survivorship as an issue to address in the **Guide to Community Preventive Services** (Truman et al., 2000). This guide provides recommendations on preventive interventions that can be used in a community setting.
- Develop tools/methods for translating research findings so that the general public can understand and apply the knowledge to their everyday life.
- Use research findings to educate cancer survivors and others (including providers, organizations, and advocates) on survivorship issues.
- Disseminate research findings to health care professionals and survivors through public health and other organizations, using a variety of venues (e.g., Internet, mail).

Section IV Summary:
Surveillance and Applied Research

1. Enhance the existing surveillance and applied research infrastructure.

2. Identify factors associated with ongoing health concerns of cancer survivors.

3. Determine programs and services that best address the needs of cancer survivors.

4. Conduct research on preventive interventions to evaluate their impact on issues related to cancer survivorship.

5. Translate applied research into practice.

Daniel, Two-time Lymphoma Survivor

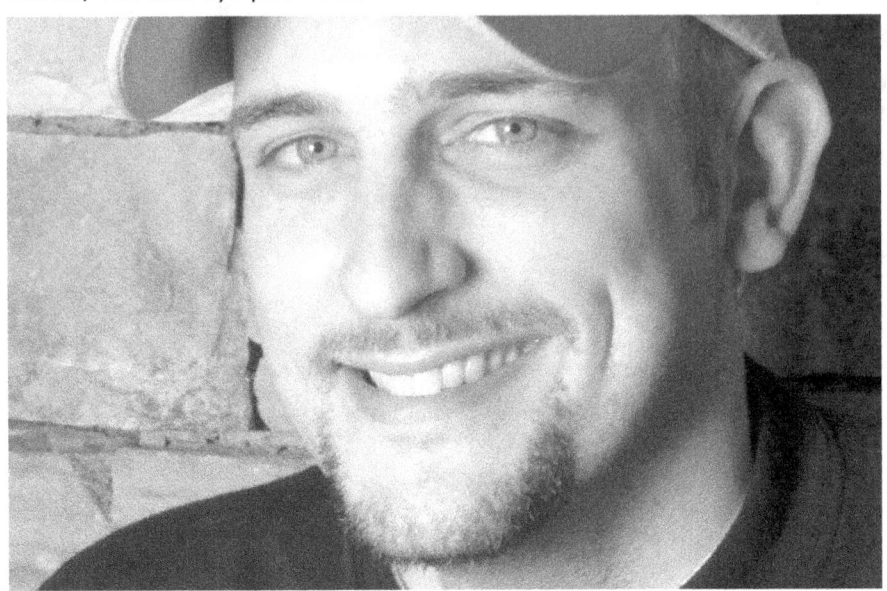

"Survivorship is far more than living through cancer treatment — it's who I am."

V. COMMUNICATION, EDUCATION, AND TRAINING

A. Goals

The ever-growing population of cancer survivors requires new information that affects not only survivors and their families but also health care providers and the public at large. These needs can be met through effective communication, education, and training efforts aimed at increasing awareness of cancer survivorship issues. These issues include the importance of effective prevention or management of secondary health concerns, appropriate management of cancer, ability to maintain adequate health coverage, adequate post-treatment care, and quality-of-life strategies for those at all stages of cancer survivorship. Goals in communication, education, and training include the following:

- Structure existing and develop new messages about cancer survivorship to reach three broad audiences: the public, cancer survivors, and health care providers.
- Tailor the content and delivery of these existing and/or developed messages for subgroups (e.g., culturally diverse groups, various health care professionals) within each of the three main audiences.
- Use factual, consistent, culturally appropriate language and information.

For the purposes of cancer survivorship, the topic areas are defined here and in Section II as follows:

Communication with the Public
Communication with the general public and policy or decision makers about the issues surrounding cancer survivorship aims to create a societal understanding and acceptance of the growing population of cancer survivors and the issues they face.

Survivor Education
Education of cancer survivors includes provision of information tailored to the particular stage of survivorship. Such educational interventions may be most appropriate during the first 5 years after diagnosis as this is the time when many of the challenges associated with the adjustment to survivorship occur (Mullan, 1984).

Provider Training
Health care provider training aims to ensure that providers are aware of the medical and other special needs of cancer survivors so they can

offer the spectrum of services available to enhance quality of life throughout survivorship and refer survivors to these services as appropriate.

Prioritized needs for these components and suggested strategies for addressing them are presented in the following section.

B. Prioritized Needs and Suggested Strategies

One aim of communication with the public is to dispel the myth that cancer is an inevitably disabling or fatal disease (Leigh & Clark, 1998). This misconception may lead to fear and discrimination that creates a difficult environment for survivors. For example, 25% of cancer survivors experience some form of employment discrimination based on their medical history (Hoffman, 1991). This may come in the form of demotions, reduction or elimination of benefits, or may manifest itself in communications or relationships with coworkers (Hoffman, 1991).

The goal of communication with the public about cancer survivorship is to create societal understanding and acceptance of issues affecting survivors. Those developing public education campaigns need to take into account variations in messages and materials relating to cancer survivorship among different segments of the population. Organizations and agencies that disseminate information about cancer survivorship could partner together in these efforts to leverage resources and ensure the consistent and efficient delivery of cancer survivorship information.

Although communication with the general public regarding cancer survivorship issues is important, cancer survivors and their families need specific information. Survivors' educational needs vary depending on their stage of survivorship. Potential areas to be addressed in survivor-focused education include issues surrounding medical care after treatment, both for the first 5 years after diagnosis and the need for long-term care and/or prevention; prevention of secondary cancers and other health concerns; physical aftereffects and complications of cancer and cancer treatment; psychological and social effects of cancer diagnosis and treatment; and practical matters, such as employment and insurance coverage. An example of educational materials designed to address such issues is the Facing Forward Series, a three-part series published by NCI, designed to educate and empower cancer survivors as they face the challenges associated with life after cancer treatment. Other publications, including numerous books, such as Lance Armstrong's *It's Not About the Bike* (Armstrong & Jenkins, 2001), provide insight into the personal side of the experience of survivorship.

Health care providers play an important role in the care of cancer survivors, not only by providing diagnostic and treatment services but also by referring survivors to services that address physical, psychosocial, and economic needs throughout the span of survivorship. In many cases, however, providers may be unaware of survivors' specific needs and how they might play a role in facilitating access to services to meet these needs. Support and education program providers need to communicate with health care providers to ensure that survivors are receiving referrals to services designed to enhance quality of life throughout the stages of cancer survivorship and address their specific needs and issues in a timely manner.

1. Develop strategies to educate the public that cancer is a chronic disease that people can and do survive.
Despite significant reductions in cancer-related mortality, myths and misinformation about a cancer diagnosis persist (e.g., "diagnosis of cancer means certain death" as in Section I.C.). Accurate, culturally appropriate information is needed to counteract these misconceptions and increase understanding and acceptance of issues affecting cancer survivors. Key strategies for addressing this need include the following:

> • Convene a Task Force to identify existing educational information, and encourage partnerships to avoid duplication of efforts in developing new educational materials.
> • Enhance a centralized information resource center, such as a clearinghouse (e.g., print, on-line), to provide access to consistent, scientifically valid, culturally appropriate health communication information.
> • Promote the centralized information resource through a variety of media, including public service announcements for television, print, and the Internet.
> • Promote the concept of survivorship as a chronic condition that people can live with and not necessarily die from.

2. Educate policy- and decision-makers about the role and value of long-term follow-up care, addressing quality-of-life issues and legal needs, and ensuring access to clinical trials and ancillary services for cancer survivors.
Acknowledgment and understanding of the long-term effects of cancer can enable survivors, caregivers, and health care providers to anticipate and deal with these effects. Increased understanding may

also enable enactment of appropriate policies to ensure that survivors receive needed follow-up care. Well-informed policy and decision makers can advocate for changes in and funding of services and additional research in these areas. Key strategies for addressing this need include the following:

- Identify potential policy and decision makers and establish mechanisms to educate them on survivorship issues.
- Catalogue and characterize existing policies in order to identify gaps in survivor needs to address.
- Identify partnerships with those with an interest in national and/or state policies.
- Develop and implement specific strategies to educate each identified policy and decision maker group (e.g., legislators; local, state, and national regulators; health service administrators; advocacy groups; community-based organizations; health-related industries; insurance industry; pharmaceutical industry).

3. Empower survivors with advocacy skills.
Cancer survivors are faced with extremely difficult medical decisions at each stage of living with, through, and beyond cancer. Because medical decisions are such important component to ongoing improvement of quality of life among cancer survivors, the topic of "informed decision making" is presented in detail in the cross-cutting section (Section III).

4. Develop, test, maintain, and promote patient navigation systems for people living with cancer.
Patient navigation systems attempt to provide a mechanism to enhance the delivery of optimum care. This need is also summarized in Section III.

5. Teach survivors how to access and evaluate available information.
Cancer-related information is available from a multitude of organizations. However, this information may be inconsistent in the message content, culturally inappropriate, and/or difficult to access. A system to evaluate the validity of available cancer survivorship information is needed that can be linked to other, reliable information sources. Key strategies for addressing this need include the following:

- Develop a standardized system to assess the adequacy of available survivorship information.

- Develop resources to assist survivors in assessing survivorship information in a variety of formats (e.g., CD-ROM, pamphlets, Web pages, video).
- Disseminate the above-mentioned resources through a variety of distribution points (e.g., medical offices, cultural or faith-based community organizations, support groups, national and local associations) and through a centralized database that can be linked to other sources of reliable information.
- Provide technical assistance to groups whose materials do not meet the established evaluation criteria (i.e., do not maintain scientific validity) and enhance the quality of materials/products.

6. Educate health care providers about cancer survivorship issues from diagnosis through long-term treatment effects and end-of-life care.

Health care providers include all clinical, community, and public health professionals who potentially affect the health and well-being of people living with cancer. Although the specific message will vary for different types of providers, all should understand the impact a cancer diagnosis has on quality of life, the common myths and misperceptions about cancer and accurate information to dispel them, prevention strategies for secondary illnesses, appropriate management strategies, referral sources (i.e., where and when to refer), sources of support, and long-term treatment effects and end-of-life care. Key strategies for addressing this need among providers include the following:

- Establish educational forums on survivorship in partnership with professional organizations.
- Educate health professionals and para-professionals in local medical communities through grand rounds, tumor board meetings, and other venues.
- Partner with advocacy groups to visit community practices and observe/educate local providers about implications of and opportunities for improving quality of life.
- Incorporate survivorship curricula into professional/para-professional training programs.
- Develop continuing education training in survivorship to deliver to a variety of health care professionals (e.g., internists, nurses).

Section V Summary: Communication, Education, and Training

1. Develop strategies to educate the public that cancer is a chronic disease people can and do survive.

2. Educate policy- and decision-makers about the role and value of long-term follow-up care, addressing quality-of-life issues and legal needs, and ensuring access to clinical trials and ancillary services for cancer survivors.

3. Empower survivors with advocacy skills.

4. Develop, test, maintain, and promote patient navigation systems for people living with cancer.

5. Teach survivors how to access and evaluate available information.

6. Educate health care providers about cancer survivorship issues from diagnosis through long-term treatment effects and end-of-life care.

Mason, Wilms' Tumor Survivor

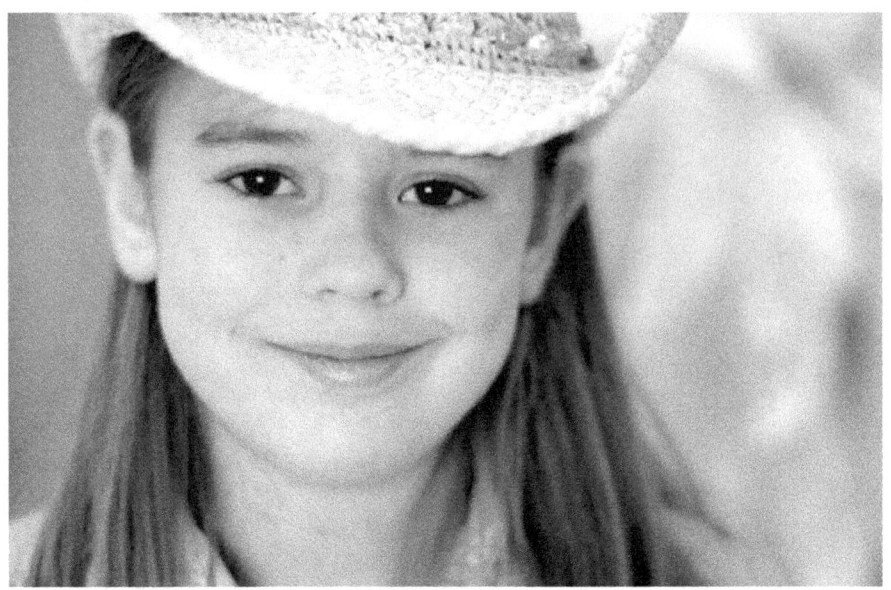

"Survivorship has shown me that cancer was really hard, but it was something I just had to go through."

VI. PROGRAMS, POLICIES, AND INFRASTRUCTURE

A. Goals

This section describes prioritized needs and recommended strategies for programs, policies, and infrastructure at national, state, and community levels to advance cancer survivorship within public health settings. Goals include the following:

- Develop a continuum of health programs and services that addresses both cancer treatment needs and primary, secondary, and tertiary prevention of additional health concerns for cancer survivors.
- Enhance supportive policies that establish an environment to comprehensively address cancer survivorship issues.
- Establish a system of services that enhances and creates partnerships among public and private health agencies.

Programs, policies, and infrastructure are means for effecting change and are defined here and in Section II.C. as follows:

Programs

Programs are the actual implementation of specific interventions at the national, state, and community levels to address a public health problem (NAAP, 1999). Medical, psychosocial, legal, and financial issues could be addressed by programs that are comprehensive in scope and encompass care for each stage of cancer survivorship.

Policies

Policies include legislation, regulations, ordinances, guidelines, and norms that establish an environment conducive to program implementation and other changes specific to survivorship (NAAP, 1999). These policies may be implemented at the national, state, organizational, and community levels in an effort to advance public health.

Infrastructure

Infrastructure is comprised of the basic resources and facilities in place to address survivorship and includes components of the health care and public health systems, such as state and local health departments, and the services and programs they provide. Effective infrastructure is required to operate and manage effective programs. As our health care system continues to evolve, delivery of quality care becomes more complex. Relationships among the public and private sectors, individual practitioners and managed care organizations, and voluntary health organizations directly influence access to care and provision of clinical and community services (NAAP, 1999).

Prioritized needs for these components and suggested strategies for addressing them are presented in the following section.

B. Prioritized Needs and Suggested Strategies

It is through programs, policies, and infrastructure that public health can effect change in terms of the delivery of services for cancer survivors. Survivorship initiatives could be embedded in all services related to the continuum of care, including cancer prevention, screening and early detection, diagnosis and treatment, rehabilitation, and palliative and end-of-life care. These programs may be offered through a variety of sources, such as comprehensive cancer centers, advocacy organizations, or community-based organizations (Tesauro et al., 2002). Policies may be implemented at the national, state, and community levels to create an environment supportive of advancing cancer survivorship in the realm of public health. An example of an existing policy that is relevant to cancer survivorship is the Cancer Survivors' Bill of Rights© (Spingarn, 1999). The Bill was written by a cancer survivor for cancer survivors and denotes the shift in a survivor's role from passive patienthood to proactivity (Leigh & Stovall, 1998). This document serves as an example of how an advocacy organization can advance policy in the realm of cancer survivorship.

Exploring ways that public health policy can be developed to address the needs of cancer survivors is an important next step in action planning. To ensure that cancer survivorship innovations reach the people who need them most, states, territories, and tribal organizations need to build and maintain appropriate infrastructure. Sufficient scientific and programmatic infrastructure will enable health agencies to build the necessary coalitions and partnerships to translate research into public health programs, practices, and services for cancer survivors. CCC Programs (see Section I.D.) hold promise as the foundation for developing this infrastructure specific to cancer prevention and control.

1. Develop, test, maintain, and promote patient navigation or case management programs that facilitate optimum care.
Patient navigation is a tool that can be used to ensure that survivors understand their care and their process of care and enhance the delivery of optimum care. In these programs, health professionals or highly trained patient liaison representatives coordinate health care

for patients and assist them in navigating the health care system. This need is discussed in detail in Section III.

2. Develop and disseminate public education programs that empower survivors to make informed decisions.
No one medical answer is right for everyone. Cancer survivors are faced with extremely difficult medical decisions at each stage of living with, through, and beyond cancer. This need is presented in Section III.

3. Identify and implement programs proven to be effective (i.e., best practices).
In the public health field, "best practices" refer to programs that have been identified as effective through a standardized process using commonly agreed-upon criteria for rating their success (USDHHS, 2003). These programs have been shown to be successful through measurable outcomes. Efforts are under way within public health to systematically identify these programs and disseminate them to a broader audience for replication (USDHHS, 2003). Within the realm of cancer survivorship, there is much to learn about the best practices of programs that address needs for people living with, through, and beyond cancer. Specific strategies to achieve the goal of identifying and disseminating best practices for cancer survivorship include the following:

- Establish quantifiable criteria to determine which programs are among the best practices for addressing cancer survivor needs.
- Identify best practices based on agreed-upon criteria and rank order programs accordingly.
- Identify gaps in survivorship research and provide funding to test new models and approaches.
- Establish a "clearinghouse" of information (e.g., **Cancer Control PLANET**, CIS) using existing mechanisms for those programs identified as best practices.
- Promote this "clearinghouse" and otherwise disseminate information to programs, survivors, health care providers, and others. Use this clearinghouse to connect survivors to resources specific to their needs.

4. Implement evidence-based cancer plans that include all stages of cancer survivorship.
Through the CDC's funding of CCC Programs (see Section I.D.), states are developing cancer control plans to comprehensively address

this disease. States launched these Programs in collaboration with private and not-for-profit entities to assure appropriate expertise and to maximize the impact of limited resources on cancer control efforts. Public health agencies are using this support to establish broad-based cancer coalitions, assess the burden of cancer, determine priorities for cancer prevention and control, and develop and implement comprehensive plans. Through these and other activities, work is under way to identify those efforts that are grounded in sound scientific knowledge, or are "evidence based." Evidence-based efforts in public health rely on a rigorous process where strategies to address a health issue are assessed to identify those with the highest quality scientific evidence of successful outcomes. Too often, rigorous evidence is lacking upon which to recommend strategies and interventions to address important goals and objectives. Most states have included issues related to cancer survivorship in their plans but have not necessarily included efforts that are evidence-based or that address needs for each stage of living with, through, and beyond cancer. There is a need to identify evidence-based initiatives that can be systematically incorporated into state cancer control efforts. The following strategies provide specific guidance to meet this need:

- Identify key leaders and experts in cancer survivorship in every state (especially survivors) to create a network of individuals to ensure that survivorship issues are being addressed through each cancer plan.
- Educate those involved in planning and developing state cancer plans on the importance of and issues related to cancer survivorship.
- Evaluate survivorship programs and publish and disseminate results.
- Link CCC Program and other funding so that cancer plans are required to comprehensively address survivorship.

5. Establish clinical practice guidelines for each stage of cancer survivorship.

Clinical practice guidelines are defined by the IOM as "...systematically developed statements to assist practitioner and patient decisions for specific clinical circumstances" (IOM, 1992). These guidelines summarize the collective research on outcomes pertaining to one disease. This need is presented in detail in Section III.

6. Promote policy changes that support addressing cancer as a long-term, chronic disease.

Historically, cancer was a disease that people often did not survive (see Section I.A.). Health care focused on making the patient comfortable during the last stages of cancer progression; few treatment options were available. Now, many more treatment options are available, and people survive with cancer for many years. The medical model tends to focus more on cancer survivors during their "acute" stages of cancer and less on the "extended" and "permanent" stages (Mullan, 1985) and not on post-treatment or long-term issues. Policies need to effectively address cancer survivorship for all those living with, through, and beyond cancer. Strategies for effecting this change include the following:

- Develop and disseminate public education materials to educate policy makers, health professionals, and survivors on the stages of cancer survivorship.
- Encourage insurance carriers and health plan administrators to provide for post-treatment and long-term follow-up services for cancer survivors.
- Address the terminology used in various settings, such as in formal policy and the media, at health care organizations and among providers and insurance agencies, to modify policies to better reflect the stages of cancer survivorship.

7. Develop infrastructure to obtain quality data on all cancer management activities to support programmatic action.

A great deal is unknown about cancer survivorship, particularly in terms of the long-term effects of cancer diagnosis and treatment. For that reason, much work needs to be done to create comprehensive databases to collect information on survivors and conduct research on issues related to survivorship. This need is discussed in detail in Section III.

Section VI Summary:
Programs, Policies, and Infrastructure

1. Develop, test, maintain, and promote patient navigation or case management programs that facilitate optimum care.

2. Develop and disseminate public education programs that empower survivors to make informed decisions.

3. Identify and implement programs proven to be effective (i.e., best practices).

4. Implement evidence-based cancer plans that include all stages of cancer survivorship.

5. Establish clinical practice guidelines for each stage of cancer survivorship.

6. Promote policy changes that support addressing cancer as a long-term, chronic disease.

7. Develop infrastructure to obtain quality data on all cancer management activities to support programmatic action.

Bart, Cancer Survivor

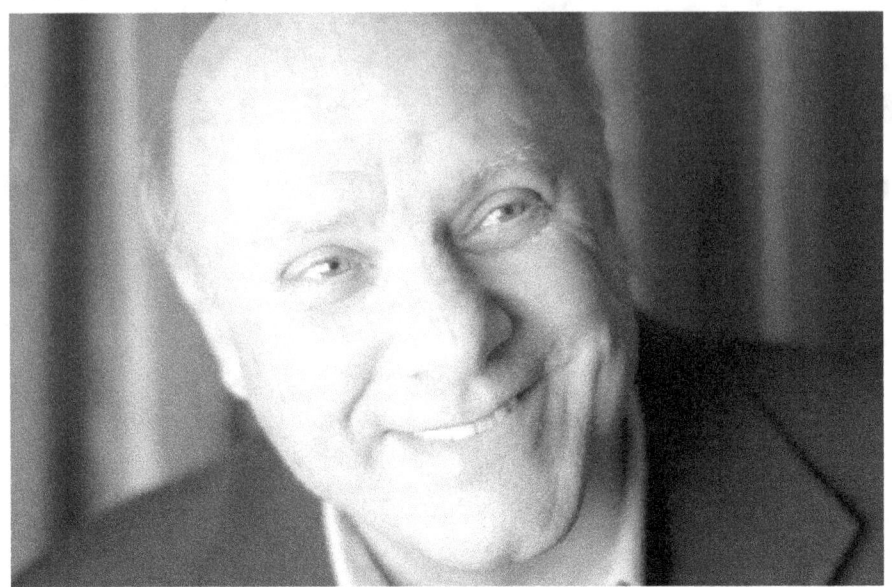

"Survivorship has given me a more complete sense of the gift of life."

VII. ACCESS TO QUALITY CARE AND SERVICES

A. Goals

This section describes prioritized needs and recommended strategies to address access to quality care and services for people living with, through, and beyond cancer. In relation to cancer survivorship, quality care and services include access to quality treatment, effective pain and symptom management, and quality end-of-life care and services. Progress in these key areas is necessary to assure quality service provision for those living with cancer. Goals in this area include the following:

- Establish clinical care guidelines to ensure availability of high-quality care for all cancer survivors.
- Provide access to high-quality care throughout every stage of cancer survivorship.
- Educate survivors on available resources and strategies to enhance informed decision making.
- Ensure coordinated care among all health care professionals involved in delivering services.

For the purposes of cancer survivorship, access to quality treatment, effective pain and symptom management, and quality end-of-life care are defined here and in Section II.C. as follows:

Access to Quality Treatment
Cancer treatment is complex and differs for each individual based on his or her specific situation and needs. All cancer survivors should have timely access to the latest and most effective treatments available. This would include clinical trials, if appropriate.

Pain and Symptom Management
An important part of cancer treatment is the management of pain and other symptoms associated with both disease and treatment. The goal of pain and symptom management is to provide relief so that survivors can tolerate the diagnostic and therapeutic procedures needed to treat their cancer and live comfortably throughout each stage of living with, through, and beyond cancer.

End-of-Life Care
Issues facing survivors and their families during end-of-life are complex and serious. Appropriate end-of-life care affirms life and regards dying as a normal process, neither hastening nor postponing death. The goal of end-of-life care is to achieve the best possible

quality of life for cancer survivors. Although many survivors live many years beyond their diagnosis, the needs and desires of those who are in the process of dying must be addressed.

Prioritized needs and suggested strategies for addressing access to quality care and services are presented in the following section.

B. Prioritized Needs and Suggested Strategies

Quality cancer care means assuring that survivors have access to evidence-based and appropriate treatment and services delivered in a timely and technically competent manner, with good communication, shared decision making, and cultural sensitivity across the continuum of care and throughout the remainder of life. Accountability is an important aspect of quality care (IOM, 1999). Health care providers must be accountable for professional competence, legal and ethical conduct, and accessibility of services (Emanuel & Emanuel, 1996).

Prioritized needs and suggested strategies to address access to quality care and services include the following:

1. Develop, test, maintain, and promote a patient navigation system for cancer survivors.

Patient navigation is a tool that can be used to ensure that survivors understand their care and their process of care as well as to enhance the delivery of optimum care. This need is described in detail in Section III.

2. Educate decision-makers about economic and insurance barriers related to health care for cancer survivors.

Survivorship advocates support the position that cancer survivors should have access to the latest and most effective treatments available and that access to these treatments should be based on the type of care needed and not on the cost of care. Unfortunately, there are many barriers to achieving this ideal of comprehensive access to quality care. The first step toward this ideal is to educate decision makers about the needs of cancer survivors and the financial barriers affecting cancer survivors' access to quality care. Strategies to help assure that decision makers are adequately informed include the following:

- Convene a meeting of health care providers, cancer survivorship experts, researchers, and programmatic staff with the goal of developing strategies to educate policy makers about the unmet needs for cancer treatment of uninsured and underinsured survivors.

- Identify successful policy and legislative language as examples for state programs (and others), and identify key stakeholders (e.g., legislators, governors) needed to improve access to high quality treatment and other post-treatment follow-up services.
- Survey and analyze the insured population to determine the impact the individual's level of coverage has on timely access to care and receipt of follow-up care.
- Develop educational opportunities for decision makers of insurance carriers and health plans regarding policies that promote access to quality cancer care.

3. Establish and/or disseminate guidelines that support quality and timely service provision to cancer survivors.
In their statement, "Principles of Quality Cancer Care," the Cancer Leadership Council emphasized that all people with cancer need to have timely access to care that is based on the best available evidence (NCCS, 2003). A key strategy for meeting this need is to develop a process for establishing clinical care guidelines for each stage of cancer survivorship. This need is discussed in detail in Section III of this National Action Plan.

4. Assess and enhance provision of palliative services to cancer survivors.
The goal of palliative care is to achieve the best possible quality of life for survivors and their families by controlling pain and other symptoms and addressing psychological and spiritual needs throughout each stage of living with, through, and beyond cancer. Strategies to assess and enhance provision of palliative services to cancer survivors include the following:

- Collect baseline **quantitative** and **qualitative data** to assess the current status and location of palliative service provision, and characterize the experiences of survivors, their caregivers, and providers in relation to palliative care.
- Provide professional and public education to teach people about palliative care, how health care providers should administer such services, and how survivors and their caregivers can advocate for this care.
- Establish regulatory policies for licensing and agency responsibility for palliative care oversight.

- Provide training for medical personnel on the topic of substance abuse to help alleviate fears of misuse of pain medications and increase professional acceptance of prescribing pain control medications to cancer survivors.
- Develop targeted therapies to manage cancer pain so that concerns about unintended consequences of pain medication administration can be avoided.

5. Establish integrated multidisciplinary teams of health care providers.

Cancer treatment is complex and differs for each individual based on his or her specific situation and needs. To assure that each cancer survivor receives appropriate and comprehensive treatment, these efforts should be planned, coordinated, and delivered by a multidisciplinary team of providers. Strategies to establish such multidisciplinary teams include the following:

- Create centers of excellence (using pediatric cancer centers as a model) that provide comprehensive care to cancer survivors especially for rarer forms of cancer.
- Formulate policies that will improve access to services provided to survivors from an appropriate provider of choice.
- Promote and provide increased access to clinical trials and longitudinal follow-up through the centers of excellence.
- Develop survivor-oriented Web sites to guide follow-up after completion of primary treatment.
- Develop mechanisms (e.g., password-protected Web forum, telephone, mail) for survivors to have ongoing routine follow-up with their multidisciplinary team after primary treatment. Follow-up should be annual at a minimum.
- Develop survivorship programs through appropriate partner organizations (e.g., the American College of Surgeons Commission on Cancer, NCCS) to provide professional education on cancer survivorship.
- Ensure survivor access to symptom management/palliative care/supportive teams.
- Review management plans from other chronic disease models (e.g., diabetes) and use these as a basis to develop integrated multidisciplinary management plans for cancer survivorship.
- Ensure that integrated multidisciplinary management is available to survivors across the continuum of care.

Section VII Summary: Access to Quality Care and Services

1. Develop, test, maintain, and promote a patient navigation system for cancer survivors.

2. Educate decision-makers about economic and insurance barriers related to health care for cancer survivors.

3. Establish and/or disseminate guidelines that support for quality and timely service provision to cancer survivors.

4. Assess and enhance provision of palliative services to cancer survivors.

5. Establish integrated multidisciplinary teams of health care providers.

Octavio, Cancer Survivor

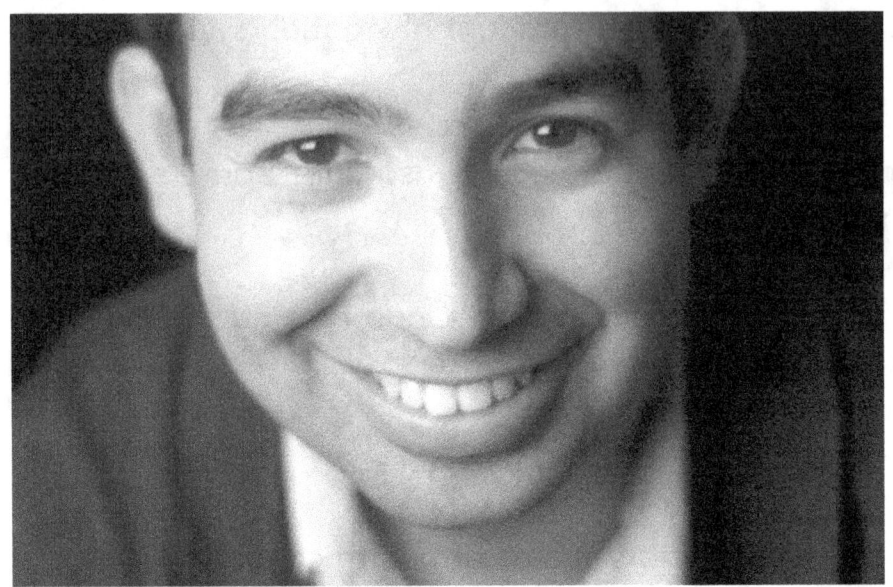

"Survivorship means coming out of my cancer experience as a whole person and being able to make it an important and positive part of who I am."

VIII. IMPLEMENTATION

A. Indicators

In order to evaluate the extent to which the long-term goals of the National Action Plan are reached, establishing and monitoring measures to demonstrate progress toward obtaining those goals are critical. Developing indicators provides a benchmark to gauge success and identify movement toward cancer survivorship objectives. Important indicators to measure include those related to process, such as whether initiatives are being delivered as planned, and outcomes, such as if the survivor's life is improving. Eventually, preliminary indicators can be made into measurable objectives as part of a comprehensive evaluation plan. Examples of some indicators that organizations or individuals could use for activities summarized in this Plan might include the following:

Surveillance and Applied Research
- Increase the number of cancer registries that are able to follow cancer survivors over time.
- Create a standardized set of items for the collection and analysis of cancer survivorship data, including quality of life, at the national level.
- Assess the feasibility of obtaining population-based cancer survivorship data using cancer registries and other data sources.
- Develop research initiatives to quantify health concerns of cancer survivors.
- Increase the number of collaborative efforts between academic researchers and state health departments related to cancer survivors.
- Determine the extent to which these collaborative efforts result in useful and applicable findings.

Communication, Education, and Training
- Increase health care professionals' and the general public's knowledge of the burden of cancer survivorship and issues faced by survivors.
- Increase the amount of media time devoted to cancer survivorship compared with other health issues.
- Increase the number of trainings on cancer survivorship for health professionals and para-professionals.

Programs, Policies, and Infrastructure

- Increase programmatic resources for cancer survivorship over a period of 5 years, and assess trends in funding levels across private and public sector programs.
- Increase the number of state cancer plans and CCC Programs with cancer survivorship components.
- Track the number of policies related to cancer survivorship at the local, state, and national level.
- Increase the number of health insurance carriers providing for post-treatment and long-term follow-up services, including specialty care, for cancer survivors.

Access to Quality Care and Services

- Increase the number of survivors receiving pain control and other support services throughout each stage of cancer survivorship, from diagnosis through end-of-life.
- Increase research to evaluate the effectiveness of patient navigation systems on improving cancer survivors' quality of life and disseminate those results to the public health community.
- Continue to improve the 5-year survival rates for all cancers.

B. Conclusion

With one-third of Americans estimated to be diagnosed with cancer in their lifetime, the individual and societal burden of cancer is clear. A National Action Plan for Cancer Survivorship: Advancing Public Health Strategies describes a variety of proven public health interventions as well as new strategies aimed to improve the quality of life for cancer survivors, their families, friends, and caregivers. By using the National Action Plan as a guide as well as a call to action, the public health community can initiate and sustain changes that will lead to improved quality of life among the millions of people living with, through, and beyond cancer. The ambitious approaches outlined in this National Action Plan will be most feasible if public health organizations and individuals pursue the strategies that are most applicable to their mission. Next steps for implementing this National Action Plan will be for organizations to prioritize the needs they can address and effectively implement initiatives so that progress over the next 5 years in advancing cancer survivorship within the realm of public health can be realized.

Liz, Cancer Survivor

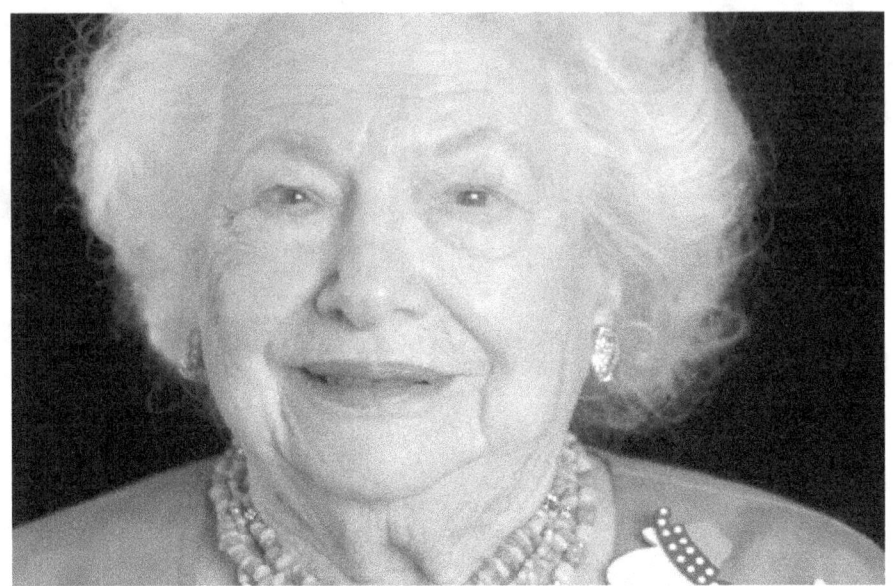

"Survivorship is life."

EXPLANATIONS OF PHRASES AND TERMS

Note: Listed below are explanations of phrases and terms that appear in the National Action Plan as bold text.

Access to quality care and services
Quality cancer care means ensuring that survivors have access to evidence-based (or proven to be successful) appropriate treatment. Services should be delivered in a timely and technically competent manner, utilizing good communication, shared decision making between the cancer survivor and health care providers, and in a cultural sensitivity manner across the continuum of care and throughout the remainder of life (IOM, 1999).

Access to quality treatment
Cancer treatment is complex and differs for each individual based on his or her specific situation and needs. Cancer survivors should have timely access to the latest and most effective treatments available. This would include clinical trials, if appropriate (Cancer Leadership Council, 2003).

Acute stage
The "acute" stage of survival begins with diagnosis and spans the time of further diagnostic and treatment efforts (Mullan, 1985).

Ancillary services
Professional services provided by a hospital or other inpatient health program. These may include x-ray, drug, laboratory, or other services (CMS, 2003).

Applied research
Use of surveillance data to better understand the extent to which interventions effectively address survivor needs and provide findings that can guide further development of initiatives.

Best practices
Programs that have been identified as effective through a standardized process using commonly agreed-upon criteria for rating their success (USDHHS, 2003).

Cancer
A term for diseases in which abnormal cells divide without control (NCI, 2003c).

Cancer Control PLANET
Plan, Link, Act, Network with Evidence-based Tools: a Web portal resource with links to resources for comprehensive cancer control (Cancer http://cancercontrolplanet.cancer.gov).

Cancer survivors
People who have been diagnosed with cancer and the people in their lives who are affected by their diagnosis, including family members, friends, and caregivers (LAF, 2003).

Case management
A process used by a doctor, nurse, or other health professional to manage a patient's health care. Case managers make sure that people receive needed services and track the use of facilities and resources (CMS, 2003).

Chronic disease
A disease that has one or more of the following characteristics: is permanent; leaves residual disability; is caused by nonreversible pathological alteration; requires special training of the patient for rehabilitation; or may be expected to require a long period of supervision, observation, or care (DEHA, 2003).

Clinical practice guidelines
Systematically developed statements designed to assist practitioner and patient decisions for specific clinical circumstances (IOM, 1992).

Clinical trials
Research studies, where patients help scientists find the best way to prevent, detect, diagnose, or treat diseases (NCI, 2003c).

Communication with the public
Communication with the general public and policy or decision makers about the issues surrounding cancer survivorship, which aims to create a societal understanding and acceptance of the growing population of cancer survivors and the issues they face.

Comprehensive cancer control
An integrated and coordinated approach to reducing cancer incidence, morbidity, and mortality through prevention (primary prevention), early detection (secondary prevention), treatment, rehabilitation, and palliation (CDC, 2003b).

End-of-life care

Affirms life and regards dying as a normal process, neither hastening nor postponing death while providing relief from distress and integrating psychological and spiritual aspects of patient care. The goal of end-of-life care is to achieve the best possible quality of life for cancer survivors by controlling pain and other symptoms and addressing psychological and spiritual needs (Hospice, 2003).

Extended stage

The "extended" stage of survival begins when the patient goes into remission or has completed treatment (Mullan, 1985).

Guide to Community Preventive Services

The Community Guide summarizes what is known about the effectiveness, economic efficiency, and feasibility of interventions to promote community health and prevent disease. The Task Force on Community Preventive Services makes recommendations for the use of various interventions based on the evidence gathered in the rigorous and systematic scientific reviews of published studies conducted by the review teams of the Community Guide. Findings from the reviews are published in peer-reviewed journals and also made available on the internet at www.thecommunityguide.org.

Health care provider

A person who is trained and licensed to give health care. Also, a place licensed to give health care. Doctors, nurses, hospitals, skilled nursing facilities, some assisted living facilities, and certain kinds of home health agencies are examples of health care providers (CMS, 2003).

Healthy People 2010

Healthy People 2010 is a set of health objectives for the nation to achieve over the first decade of the new century. It can be used by many different people, states, communities, professional organizations, and others to help them develop programs to improve health (USDHHS, 2003).

Incidence

The number of new cases of a disease diagnosed each year (NCI, 2003c).

Indicator

A substitute measure for a concept that is not directly observable or measurable (e.g., prejudice, substance abuse). Also defined as a variable that relates directly to some part of a program goal or objective. Positive change on an indicator is presumed to indicate progress in accomplishing the larger program objective (PSAP, 2003).

Infrastructure

The systems, competencies, relationships, data and information systems, skilled workforce, effective public health organizations, resources, and research that enable performance of the essential public health services in every community (USDHHS, 2000).

In-kind

Contributions or assistance in a form other than money. Equipment, materials, or services of recognized value that are offered in lieu of cash (UCLA, 2003).

Living "beyond" cancer

Refers to post-treatment and long-term survivorship (LAF, 2003).

Living "through" cancer

Refers to the extended stage following treatment (LAF, 2003).

Living "with" cancer

Refers to the experience of receiving a cancer diagnosis and any treatment that may follow (LAF, 2003).

Lymphedema

A condition in which excess fluid collects in tissue and causes swelling. It may occur in the arm or leg after lymph vessels or lymph nodes in the underarm or groin are removed or treated with radiation (NCI, 2003c).

Metastasis

The spread of cancer from one part of the body to another. A tumor formed from cells that have spread is called a secondary tumor, a metastatic tumor, or a metastasis. The plural form of metastasis is metastases. Metastasized means to spread by metastasis (NCI, 2003c).

Morbidity

A disease or the incidence of disease within a population. Morbidity also refers to adverse effects caused by a treatment (NCI, 2004).

Pain and symptom management

Pain and symptom management refers to the provision of pain relief so that patients can tolerate the diagnostic and therapeutic procedures needed to treat their cancer (Foley, 1999).

Palliative care
Care given to improve the quality of life of patients who have a serious or life-threatening disease. Also called comfort care, supportive care, and symptom management (NCI, 2003c).

Patient navigation
A tool that can be used to ensure that survivors understand their care and their process of care and enhance optimum care. In these programs, health professionals and others coordinate health care for patients and assist them in navigating the health care system (http://deainfo.nci.nih.gov/advisory/pcp/video-summary.htm).

Permanent stage
The "permanent" stage is defined as a time when the "activity of the disease or likelihood of its return is sufficiently small that the cancer can now be considered permanently arrested" (Mullan, 1985, p. 272).

Policies
Policies include legislation, regulations, ordinances, guidelines, and norms that establish an environment conducive to program implementation (NAAP, 1999).

Preventive interventions
Programs, activities, and services that identify areas of behavior that can be changed to reduce cancer recurrence or increase control and promote healthy lifestyles.

Primary prevention
Measures designed to combat risk factors for illness before an illness ever has a chance to develop (McGraw-Hill, 2003).

Programs
Programs are the actual implementation of specific interventions at the national, state, and community levels to address a public health problem (NAAP, 1999).

Provider training
Health care provider training aims to assure that providers are aware of the spectrum of services available to enhance quality of life throughout survivorship so that they may refer survivors to these services as appropriate.

Public health
Public health practice is the science and art of preventing disease, prolonging life, and promoting health and well-being (Winslow, 1923). The Institute of Medicine (IOM) has defined the mission of

public health as assuring conditions in which people can be healthy (1988). Public health's mission is achieved through the application of health promotion and disease prevention technologies and interventions designed to improve and enhance quality of life (PHFSC, 1994).

Qualitative data
A record of thoughts, observations, opinions, or words gathered/collected from open-ended questions to which the answers are not limited by a set of choices or a scale (PSAP, 2003).

Quantitative data
Numeric information that includes such items as type of treatment, amount of time, or a rating of an opinion on a scale from 1 to 5. Quantitative data are collected through closed-ended questions, where users are given a limited set of possible answers to a question (PSAP, 2003).

Risk
The probability that an event will occur (e.g., that an individual will become ill or die within a stated period of time or age) (Last, 1995).

Risk factor
Something that may increase the chance of developing a disease. Some examples of risk factors for cancer include age, a family history of certain cancers, use of tobacco products, certain eating habits, obesity, exposure to radiation or other cancer-causing agents, and certain genetic changes (NCI, 2003c).

Stakeholders
A stakeholder is someone who has a stake in an organization or a program. Stakeholders either affect the organization/program or are affected by it (PSAP, 2003).

Surveillance
Primary surveillance measures include cancer registries and several national surveys. Cancer registries implement and maintain information systems designed to collect and manage data on cases of cancer incidence. National surveys, such as the National Health Interview Survey (NHIS), provide information on health attitudes, beliefs, and behaviors that could be used to help understand issues related to cancer survivorship (CDC, 2003b).

Survivor education
The education of cancer survivors includes provision of information tailored to the particular stage of survivorship (Mullan, 1984).

REFERENCES

American Cancer Society (ACS). *Cancer Facts & Figures 2004.* Atlanta, GA: American Cancer Society; 2004.

Armstrong L, Jenkins S. *It's Not About the Bike: My Journey Back to Life.* Berkeley, CA: Berkley Publishing Group; 2001.

Aziz N. Cancer survivorship research: challenge and opportunity. *The Journal of Nutrition.* 2002;132(11):3494S-3503S.

Aziz NM, Rowland JH. Trends and advances in cancer survivorship research: challenge and opportunity. *Seminars in Radiation Oncology.* 2003;13:248-266.

Cancer Leadership Council. *CLC Mission* [on-line]. Available at: http://www.cancerleadership.org/about_clc/mission.html; Accessed November 17, 2003.

Centers for Disease Control and Prevention (CDC). Framework for program evaluation in public health. *Morbidity and Mortality Weekly Report.* 1999;48(RR11):1-40.

Centers for Disease Control and Prevention (CDC). *National Program of Cancer Registries—State/Territory Profiles* [on-line]. Atlanta, GA: U.S. Department of Health and Human Services, Centers for Disease Control and Prevention. Available at: http://www.cdc.gov/cancer/dbdata.htm; 2001.

Centers for Disease Control and Prevention (CDC). *Comprehensive Cancer Control Fact Sheet* [on-line]. Atlanta, GA: U.S. Department of Health and Human Services, Centers for Disease Control and Prevention. Available at: http://www.cdc.gov/ cancer/ncccp/about.htm; 2002.

Centers for Disease Control and Prevention (CDC). *Cancer Prevention and Control: About the Program* [on-line]. Atlanta, GA: U.S. Department of Health and Human Services, Centers for Disease Control and Prevention. Available at: http://www.cdc.gov/ cancer/dcpc.htm; 2003a.

Centers for Disease Control and Prevention. *Glossary* [on-line]. Available at: http://www.cdc.gov/tobacco/evaluation_manual/glossary.html; 2003b.

Centers for Medicare & Medicaid Services. *Glossary* [on-line]. Available at: http://www.cms.hhs.gov/glossary/default.asp; Accessed November 17, 2003.

Delaware Health Care Association (DEHA). *Glossary of Health Care Terms* [on-line]. Available at: www.deha.org/Glossary/GlossaryC.htm; Accessed November 17, 2003.

Emanuel EJ, Emanuel LL. What is accountability in health care? *Annals of Internal Medicine.* 1996;124(2):229-239.

Foley KM. Advances in cancer pain. *Archives of Neurology.* 1999;56:413-417.

Hoffman B. Employment discrimination: another hurdle for cancer survivors. *Cancer Investigation.* 1991;9:589-595.

Hospice. *What is Hospice?* [on-line]. Available at: http://www.hospicefoundation.org/what_is/; Accessed November 17, 2003.

Institute of Medicine (IOM), Committee for the Study of the Future of Public Health, Division of Health Care Services. *The Future of Public Health.* Washington, DC: National Academy Press; 1988.

Institute of Medicine (IOM). *Guidelines for Clinical Practice: From Development to Use*. Field MJ, Lohr KN, eds. Washington, DC: National Academy Press. Available at: http://www.nap.edu/openbook/0309045894/html/R1.html; 1992.

Institute of Medicine (IOM). *Approaching Death: Improving Care at the End of Life*. Field MJ, Cassel CK, eds. Washington, DC: National Academy Press; 1997.

Institute of Medicine (IOM) and Commission on Life Sciences (CLS). *Ensuring Quality Cancer Care*. Hewitt M, Simone JV, eds. Washington, DC: National Academy Press; 1999.

Institute of Medicine (IOM). *Childhood Cancer Survivorship: Improving Care and Quality of Life*. Washington, DC: National Academy Press; 2003.

Lance Armstrong Foundation. LAF [on-line]. Available at: http://www.laf.org/; Accessed November 17, 2003.

Leigh SA, Stovall EL. Cancer survivorship quality of life. In: King CR, Hinds PS, eds. *Quality of Life from Nursing and Patient Perspectives: Theory, Research*. Sudbury, MA: Jones and Bartlett Publishers; 1998:287-300.

Leigh SA, Clark EJ. Psychosocial aspects of cancer survivorship. In: Berger A, Portenoy RK, Weissman DE, eds. *Principles and Practice of Supportive Oncology*. Philadelphia, PA: Lippincott-Raven; 1998:909-917.

Leigh SA. Defining our destiny. In: Hoffman B, ed. *A Cancer Survivor's Almanac: Charting the Journey*. Minneapolis, MN: Chronimed Publishing; 1996:261-271.

McGraw-Hill. *Health Psychology Glossary* [on-line]. Available at: highered.mcgraw-hill.com/sites/0072412976/student_view0/chapter3/glossary.html; Accessed November 17, 2003.

Mullan F. Re-entry: the educational needs of the cancer survivor. *Health Education Quarterly*. 1984;10(Spec Suppl):88-94.

Mullan F. Seasons of survival: reflections of a physician with cancer. *New England Journal of Medicine*. 1985;313:270-273.

Mulley AG. Improving the quality of decision making. *Journal of Clinical Outcomes Management*. 1995;2:9-10.

National Arthritis Action Plan: A Public Health Strategy (NAAP). Arthritis Foundation, Association of State and Territorial Health Officials, & CDC. Available at: http://www.cdc.gov/nccdphp/pdf/naap.pdf;1999.

National Cancer Institute (NCI). *Young People with Cancer: A Handbook for Parents*. Publication No. 01-2378; 2001.

National Cancer Institute (NCI). *Facing Forward Series: Life after Cancer Treatment*. Publication No. 02-2424; 2002.

National Cancer Institute (NCI). *Cancer Control and Population Sciences: Research Findings* [on-line]. Available at: http://dccps.nci.nih.gov/ocs/prevalence/index.html; 2003a.

National Cancer Institute (NCI). *Cancer.gov—What you need to know about cancer—an overview* [on-line]. Available at: http://www.cancer.gov/cancerinfo/wyntk/overview; 2003b.

National Cancer Institute (NCI). *Glossary* [on-line]. Available at: http://oesi.nci.nih.gov/aboutbc/glossary.html; 2003c.

National Cancer Institute (NCI). *Cancer.gov-Dictionary* [on-line]. Available at: http://www.nci.nih.gov/dictionary;2004.

National Coalition for Cancer Survivorship (NCCS). *Introduction to Advocacy* [on-line]. Available at: http://www.cansearch.org/policy; Accessed September 17, 2003.

National Institutes of Health (NIH). *NIH: About: NIH Almanac: Organization: National Cancer Institute* [on-line]. Available at: http://www.nih.gov/about/almanac/organization/NCI.htm; 2003.

Partners for Substance Abuse Prevention (PSAP). *Glossary of Terms* [on-line]. Available at: http://preventionpartners.samhsa.gov/resources_glossary_p2.asp; Accessed November 17, 2003.

Public Health Functions Steering Committee (PHFSC). *What is Public Health?* [on-line]. Available at: http://www.asph.org/document.cfm?page=300; 1994. Accessed April 22, 2003.

Spingarn ND. *Cancer Survivor's Bill of Rights*. Silver Spring, MD: National Coalition for Cancer Survivorship; 1999.

Task Force on Community Preventive Services (TFCPS). *Community Guide—Topic* [on-line]. Available at: http://www.thecommunityguide.org/overview/default.htm; Accessed November 17, 2003.

Tesauro GM, Rowland JH, Lustig C. Survivorship resources for post-treatment cancer survivors. *Cancer Practice*. 2002;10(6):277-283.

Truman BI, Smith-Akin CK, Hinman AR, et al. Developing the *Guide to Community Preventive Services*—overview and rationale. American Journal of Preventive Medicine. 2000;18(1S):18-26.

University of California, Los Angeles (UCLA). *UCLA Sponsored Research Glossary* [on-line]. Available at: www.research.ucla.edu/sr2/gloss.htm; Accessed November 17, 2003.

U.S. Department of Health and Human Services (USDHHS). *Healthy People 2010: Understanding and Improving Health*. 2nd ed. Washington, DC: U.S. Government Printing Office; November 2000.

U.S. Department of Health and Human Services (USDHHS). *Best Practice Initiative* [on-line]. Available at: http://phs.os.dhhs.gov/ophs/BestPractices/default.htm; 2003.

U.S. Department of Health and Human Services (USDHHS). *What is Healthy People?* [on-line]. Available at: http://www.healthypeople.gov/About/whatis.htm; Accessed November 17, 2003.

Winslow CEA. *The Evolution and Significance of the Modern Public Health Campaign*. New Haven: Yale University Press; 1923.

APPENDIX A: PARTICIPATING PARTNERS AND REVIEWERS

Carla S. Alexander
National Hospice & Palliative Care Organization
1700 Diagonal Road, Suite 625
Alexandria, VA 22314
Phone: (410) 328-7129
Fax: (410) 328-4430
E-mail: calexand@medicine.umaryland.edu

Noreen Aziz
National Cancer Institute
6130 Executive Plaza North
Rockville, MD 20852
Phone: (301) 496-0598
Fax: (301) 594-5070
E-mail: na45f@nih.gov

Mark S. Baptiste
New York State Department of Health
Rm 515 Corning Tower
Albany, NY 12237-0675
Phone: (518) 474-0512
Fax: (518) 473-2853
E-mail: msb02@health.state.ny.us

Catherine Bartlett
Lance Armstrong Foundation
P.O. Box 161150
Austin, TX 78716
Phone: (512) 236-8820, ext. 122
Fax: (512) 236-8482
E-mail: catherine@laf.org

Carol Moody Becker
U.S. Conference of Mayors
1620 I Street, NW, 4th Floor
Washington, DC 20006
Phone: (202) 328-3340
Fax: (202) 328-3361
E-mail: becker@hers.com

Nora Beidler
American Society of Clinical Oncology
1900 Duke Street, Suite 200
Alexandria, VA 22314
Phone: (703) 797-1917
Fax: (703) 684-8618
E-mail: beidlern@asco.org

Kim Belloni
Centers for Disease Control and Prevention
2858 Woodcock Boulevard
Atlanta, GA 30341
Phone: (770) 488-3011
Fax: (770) 488-4760
E-mail: ksa1@cdc.gov

Fayruz Benyousef
1020 Balanced Rock Place
Rock Round, TX 78681
Phone: (512) 476-9051, ext. 114
Fax: (512) 472-3073
E-mail: fayruz@balletaustin.org

Jennifer A. Biggy
Congressman Roger Wicker's Office
2455 Rayburn House Office Building
Washington, DC 20515
Phone: (202) 225-4306
Fax: (202) 225-3549
E-mail: jennifer.biggy@mail.house.gov

Edward Billings
American Cancer Society
901 E Street, NW, Suite 500
Washington, DC 20004
Phone: (202) 661-5720
Fax: (202) 661-5750
E-mail: ted.billings@cancer.org

Bruce L. Black
American Cancer Society
1599 Clifton Road, NE
Atlanta, GA 30329
Phone: (404) 329-7716
Fax: (404) 325-2548
E-mail: bblack@cancer.org

Donald K. Blackman
Centers for Disease Control and Prevention
4770 Buford Highway, NE, MS K55
Atlanta, GA 30341
Phone: (770) 488-3023
Fax: (770) 488-4639
E-mail: dblackman@cdc.gov

Dianah C. Bradshaw
North Carolina Division of Health & Human Services
1915 Mail Service Center
Raleigh, NC 27699-1915
Phone: (919) 715-0119
Fax: (919) 715-3153
E-mail: Dianah.Bradshaw@ncmail.net

Jubilee Brown
University of Texas, M.D. Anderson Cancer Center
1515 Holcombe Blvd., Box 440
Houston, TX 77030
Phone: (713) 792-9599
Fax: (713) 792-7586
E-mail: jurobinso@mdanderson.org

Joanna Bull
Gilda's Club Worldwide
P.O. Box 297
Rensselaerville, NY 12147
Phone: (518) 797-5255
E-mail: Joanna_bull@yahoo.com

Rita M. Butterfield
Dana-Farber Cancer Institute
44 Binney Street
Boston, MA 02115
Phone: (617) 632-2182
Fax: (617) 632-4858
E-mail: rita_butterfield@dfci.harvard.edu

Molly F. Cade
Ovarian Cancer National Alliance
6444 10th Street, SE
Prior Lake, MN 55372
Phone: (952) 890-8775
E-mail: mfcade@integraonline.com

Carol Callaghan
Michigan Department of Community Health
3423 N. Martin Luther King Blvd.
Lansing, MI 48906
Phone: (517) 335-9616
Fax: (517) 335-9397
E-mail: callaghanc@michigan.gov

Erie E. Calloway
Sisters Network, Incorporated
8787 Woodway Drive, Suite 4206
Houston, TX 77063
Phone: (713) 781-0255
Fax: (713) 780-8998
E-mail: sisnet4@aol.com

Laura Caisley
Centers for Disease Control and Prevention
4770 Buford Highway, NE
Atlanta, GA 30341
Phone: (770) 488-3021
Fax: (770) 488-4760
E-mail: LCaisley@cdc.gov

Ellen E. Casey
Dana-Farber Cancer Institute
44 Binney Street, D326
Boston, MA 02115
Phone: (617) 632-2910
Fax: (617) 632-2473
E-mail: ellen_casey@dfci.harvard.edu

Katie Clarke
Sonnenschein Nath & Rosenthal
1301 K Street, NW, Suite 500
Washington, DC 20005
Phone: (202) 408-6445
Fax: (202) 408-6399
E-mail: kclarke@sonnenschein.com

Janet Collins
Centers for Disease Control and Prevention
4770 Buford Highway, NE, MS K-40
Atlanta, GA 30341
Phone: (770) 488-5402
Fax: (770) 488-5971
E-mail: jlc1@cdc.gov

George Dahlman
The Leukemia & Lymphoma Society
11 Canal Centre #111
Alexandria, VA 22314
Phone: (703) 535-6650 ext. 15
Fax: (703) 535-8163
E-mail: dahlmang@southern.leukemia-lymphoma.org

Beth Darnley
Patient Advocate Foundation
700 Thimble Shoals Boulevard, Suite 200
Newport News, VA 23606
Phone: (800) 532-5274
Fax: (757) 873-8999
E-mail: bethd@patientadvocate.org

Angelina Esparza
University of Texas, M.D. Anderson Cancer Center
1515 Holcombe Boulevard
Houston, TX 77009
Phone: (713) 792-3357
Fax: (713) 796-8347
E-mail: aesparza@mdanderson.org

Tiffany Galligan
Lance Armstrong Foundation
P.O. Box 161150
Austin, TX 78716
Phone: (512) 236-8820, ext. 128
E-mail: tiffany@laf.org

Angela Geiger
American Cancer Society
1599 Clifton Road, NE
Atlanta, GA 30329
Phone: (404) 327-6414
Fax: (404) 325-9341
E-mail: ageiger@cancer.org

Hellen Gelband
Institute of Medicine
500 5th Street, NW, #733
Washington, DC 20001
Phone: (202) 334-1446
Fax: (202) 334-2647
E-mail: Hgelband@nas.edu

Alisa M. Gilbert
The National Office of Native Cancer Survivorship
13790 Davis Street
Anchorage, AK 99516
Phone: (800) 315-8848
Fax: (907) 333-2071
E-mail: sulook@aol.com

Timothy J. Gilbert
Alaska Native Tribal Health Consortium
4141 Ambassador Drive
Anchorage, AK 99508
Phone: (907) 729-1916
Fax: (907) 729-1901
E-mail: tjgilbert@anthc.org

Sue A. Gilman
The Susan G. Komen Breast Cancer Foundation
7221 Brookcove Lane
Dallas, TX 75214
Phone: (214) 824-6837
Fax: (214) 824-0824
E-mail: jbgilma@attglobal.net

Leslie S. Given
Centers for Disease Control and Prevention
4770 Buford Highway, NE, MS K-57
Atlanta, GA 30341
Phone: (770) 488-3099
Fax: (770) 488-3230
E-mail: lgiven@cdc.gov

Betsy Goldberg
Lance Armstrong Foundation
P.O. Box 161150
Austin, TX 78716
Work: (512) 236-8820
Fax: (512) 236-8482
E-mail: betsy@laf.org

Karen Greendale
New York State Department of Health
Riverview Center, 3rd Floor West,
150 Broadway
Albany, NY 12204
Phone: (518) 474-1222
Fax: (518) 473-0642
E-mail: kxg03@health.state.ny.us

Ellen R. Gritz
University of Texas, M.D. Anderson Cancer Center
1515 Holcombe Boulevard, Suite 243
Houston, TX 77030-4009
Phone: (713) 792-0919
Fax: (713) 794-4730
E-mail: egritz@mdanderson.org

Susan E. Grober
Cancer Care Incorporated
275 Seventh Avenue
New York, NY 10001
Phone: (212) 712-6165
Fax: (212) 712-8495
E-mail: sgrober@cancercare.org

Wendy S. Harpham
Presbyterian Hospital of Dallas
P.O. Box 835574
Richardson, TX 75083-5574
Phone: (972) 702-0321
Fax: (972) 702-0321
E-mail: harpham@comcast.net

Amy Harris
Centers for Disease Control and Prevention
4770 Buford Highway, NE
Atlanta, GA 30341
Phone: (770) 488-4260
Fax: (770) 488-4760
E-mail: ABHarris@cdc.gov

Catherine D. Harvey
National Coalition for Cancer Survivorship
655 Cain Drive
Mt. Pleasant, SC 29464
Phone: (843) 881-4645
Fax: (843) 971-1310
E-mail: catherineharvey@comcast.net

Pamela J. Haylock
University of Texas Medical Branch
School of Nursing
18954 State Hwy 16 North
Medina, TX 78055
Phone: (830) 589-7380
Fax: (830) 589-7381
E-mail: pjhaylock@indian-creek.net

Debra J. Holden
RTI International
3040 Cornwallis Road
Research Triangle Park, NC 27709
Phone: (919) 541-6000
Fax: (919) 541-7148
E-mail: debra@rti.com

Melissa M. Hudson
St. Jude Children's Research Hospital
332 North Lauderdale Street
Memphis, TN 38105
Phone: (901) 495-3445
Fax: (901) 495-3058
E-mail: melissa.hudson@stjude.org

Linda A. Jacobs
University of Pennsylvania Abramson Cancer Center
14 Penn Tower, 3400 Spruce Street
Philadelphia, PA 19104
Phone: (215) 615-3371
Fax: (610) 615-3349
E-mail: linda.jacobs@uphs.upenn.edu

Mickey L. Jacobs
Texas Cancer Council
211 E. 7th, Suite 710
Austin, TX 78701
Phone: (512) 463-3190
Fax: (512) 475-2563
E-mail: mjacobs@tcc.state.tx.us

Harriet Jett
Centers for Disease Control and Prevention
4770 Buford Highway, NE, MS K-40
Atlanta, GA 30341
Phone: (770) 488-6472
Fax: (770) 488-5971
E-mail: hjett@cdc.gov

Stuart J. Kaplan
Children's Oncology Camp Foundation
P.O. Box 1450
Missoula, MT 59801
Phone: (901) 495-4776
Fax: (901) 495-3058
E-mail: stuart.kaplan@stjude.org

Susan L. Lamb
Oklahoma State Department of Health
Chronic Disease Services
1000 N.E.10th
Oklahoma City, OK 73117
Phone: (405) 271-4072, ext. 57126
Fax: (405) 271-5181
E-mail: susanl@health.state.ok.us

Nancy Lee
Centers for Disease Control and Prevention
2858 Woodcock Boulevard
Atlanta, GA 30341
Phone: (770) 488-3011
Fax: (770) 488-4760
E-mail: nclee@cdc.gov

Susan Leigh
National Coalition for Cancer Survivorship
505 E. Golder Ranch Road
Tuscan, AZ 85739
Phone: (520) 825-0058
Fax: (520) 825-8650
E-mail: sleigh@mindspring.com

Maureen T. Lilly
RAND Corporation
4200 Wisconsin Avenue, NW, 4th Floor
Washington, DC 20016
Phone: (202) 895-2618
Fax: (202) 966-5410
E-mail: mlilly@rand.org

Steven E. Lipshultz
University of Miami
Coral Gables, FL 33124
Phone: (305) 284-2211
E-mail: steve_lipshultz@miami.edu

Randall Macon
Lance Armstrong Foundation
P.O. Box 161150
Austin, TX 78716
Phone: (512) 236-8820
Fax: (512) 236-8482

Doug McCormack
Sonnenschein Nath & Rosenthal
1301 K Street, NW, Suite 600 East Tower
Washington, DC 20005
Phone (202) 408-9138
E-mail: dmccormack@sonnenschein.com

Anna T. Meadows
Children's Hospital of Philadelphia
34th Street & Civic Center Boulevard
Philadelphia, PA 19104
Phone: (215) 590-2804
Fax: (215) 590-4183
E-mail: meadows@email.chop.edu

Margo Michaels
National Cancer Institute, NIH
6116 Executive Boulevard, Suite 202
Rockville, MD 20892-8334
Phone: (301) 594-8993
E-mail: micham@mail.nih.gov

Susan Murchie
RTI International
3040 Cornwallis Road
Research Triangle Park, NC 27709
Phone: (919) 485-2604
Fax : (919) 541-6683
E-mail: murchie@rti.org

Donna Nichols
Texas Department of Health
350 Young School House Road
Smithville, TX 78957
Phone: (512) 458-7261
E-mail: donna.nichols@tdh.state.tx.us

Kevin C. Oeffinger
University of Texas Southwestern Medical Center
6263 Harry Hines Boulevard
Dallas, TX 75390-9067
Phone: (214) 648-1399
Fax: (214) 648-1307
E-mail: kevin.oeffinger@utsouthwestern.edu

Karen Parker
President's Cancer Panel
31 Center Drive
Building 31, Room 4A48
Bethesda, MD 20814
Phone: (301) 496-1148
Fax: (301) 402-1508
E-mail: klparker@mail.nih.gov

Marilyn M. Patterson
Oncology Nursing Society
300 Jeff Woodfin Road
Inman, SC 29349
Phone: (864) 473-2098
Fax: (864) 473-2275
E-mail: fatiguelady@hotmail.com

Diane F. Perlmutter
Gilda's Club Worldwide
322 Eighth Avenue
New York, NY 10001
Phone: (917) 305-1200, ext. 230
Fax: (917) 305-0549
E-mail: dperlmutter@gildasclub.org

Loria Pollack
Centers for Disease Control and Prevention
4700 Buford Hwy, NE, MS K-55
Atlanta, GA 30033
Phone: (770) 488-3181
Fax: (770) 488-4639
E-mail: lop5@cdc.gov

Tabatha Powell
Centers for Disease Control and Prevention
4770 Buford Highway, NE
Atlanta, GA 30341
Phone: (770) 448-4263
Fax: (770) 488-4760
E-mail: tdo3@cdc.gov

Elizabeth Randall-David
Center for Creative Education
1019 W. Markham Avenue
Durham, NC 27701
Phone: (919) 687-0886
Fax: (919) 687-0886
E-mail: Brdcfce@aol.com

Christopher J. Recklitis
Dana-Farber Cancer Institute
44 Binney Street
Boston, MA 02115
Phone: (617) 632-3839
E-mail: christopher_recklitis@dfci.harvard.edu

Leslie L. Robison
University of Minnesota
420 Delaware Street, SE, MMC 422
Minneapolis, MN 55455
Phone: (612) 626-2902
Fax: (612) 626-4842
E-mail: robison@epi.umn.edu

Phyllis Rochester
Centers for Disease Control and Prevention
4770 Buford Highway, NE
Atlanta, GA 30341
Phone: (770) 488-3096
Fax: (770) 488-3230
E-mail: pfr5@cdc.gov

Michael Samuelson
The National Center for Health Promotion
2232 S. Main Street, #475
Ann Arbor, MI 48103
Phone: (734) 429-3065
Fax: (734) 429-8309
E-mail: Michael@thenationalcenter.com

Jay L. Silver
Intercultural Cancer Council
6655 Travis Street, Suite 322
Houston, TX 77030-1312
Phone: (713) 798-1069
Fax: (713) 798-6222
E-mail: jsilver@bcm.tmc.edu

Priya Sircar
Lance Armstrong Foundation
P.O. Box 161150
Austin, TX 78716
Phone: (512) 236-8820
Fax: (512) 236-8482

Cynthia S. Soloe
RTI International
3040 Cornwallis Road
Research Triangle Park, NC 27709
Phone: (919) 541-6000
Fax: (919) 541-7148
E-mail: csoloe@rti.org

George-Ann Stokes
Centers for Disease Control and Prevention
4770 Buford Highway, NE, MS K-57
Atlanta, GA 30341
Phone: (770) 488-4780
Fax: (770) 488-3230
E-mail: gas7@cdc.gov

Ellen Stovall
National Coalition for Cancer Survivorship
1010 Wayne Avenue, Suite 770
Silver Spring, MD 20910
Phone: (301) 650-9127
Fax: (301) 565-9670
E-mail: estovall@canceradvocacy.org

Edward L. Trimble
National Cancer Institute, NIH
6130 Executive Boulevard, Suite 7025
Rockville, MD 20892-7436
Phone: (301) 496-2522
Fax: (301) 402-0557
E-mail: tt6m@nih.gov

Susan True
Centers for Disease Control and Prevention
4770 Buford Highway, NE, MS K-57
Atlanta, GA 30314
Phone: (770) 488-4880
Fax: (770) 488-3230
E-mail: smt7@cdc.gov

PerStephanie Thompson
Centers for Disease Control and Prevention
4770 Buford Highway, NE
Atlanta, GA 30341
Phone: (770) 488-4263
Fax: (770) 488-4760
E-mail: PThompson@cdc.gov

Diana Ulman
Maryland Cancer Plan
4240 Blue Barrow Ride
Ellicott City, MD 21042
Phone: (410) 461-3400
Fax: (410) 461-3401
E-mail: dulman@connext.net

Doug Ulman
Lance Armstrong Foundation
P.O. Box 161150
Austin, TX 78716
Phone: (512) 236-8820
Fax: (512) 236-8482
E-mail: doug@laf.org

Kirk Watson
Former Mayor of Austin
106 East Sixth Street, Suite 700
Austin, TX 78701
Phone: (512) 479-5900
Fax: (512) 479-5934
E-mail: Kwatson@watsonbishop.com

Fran Wheeler
Chronic Disease Directors
1107 Rutland Drive
West Columbia, SC 29169
Phone: (803) 796-9574
Fax: (803) 796-6510
E-mail: fran-wheeler@sc.rr.com

Brock Yetso
Ulman Cancer Fund for Young Adults
5575 Sterrett Place, Suite 340A
Columbia, MD 21044
Phone: (410) 964-0202
Fax: (410) 964-0402
E-mail: brock@ulmanfund.org

Joan Levy Zlotnik
Institute for the Advancement of Social Work Research
750 First Street, NE, Suite 700
Washington, DC 20002-4241
Phone: (202) 336-8393
Fax: (202) 336-8351
E-mail: jzlotnik@naswdc.org

APPENDIX B: HEALTHY PEOPLE 2010 CANCER OBJECTIVES

1. Reduce the overall cancer death rate.
2. Reduce the lung cancer death rate.
3. Reduce the breast cancer death rate.
4. Reduce the death rate from cancer of the uterine cervix.
5. Reduce the colorectal cancer death rate.
6. Reduce the oropharyngeal cancer death rate.
7. Reduce the prostate cancer death rate.
8. Reduce the rate of melanoma cancer deaths.
9. Increase the proportion of persons who use at least one of the following protective measures that may reduce the risk of skin cancer: avoid the sun between 10 a.m. and 4 p.m., wear sun-protective clothing when exposed to sunlight, use sunscreen with a sun-protective factor (SPF) of 15 or higher, and avoid artificial sources of ultraviolet light.
9a. (Developmental) Increase the proportion of adolescents in grades 9 through 12 who follow protective measures that may reduce the risk of skin cancer.
9b. Increase the proportion of adults aged 18 years and older who follow protective measures that may reduce the risk of skin cancer.
10. Increase the proportion of physicians and dentists who counsel their at-risk patients about tobacco use cessation, physical activity, and cancer screening.
11. Increase the proportion of women who receive a Pap test.
12. Increase the proportion of adults who receive a colorectal cancer screening examination
13. Increase the proportion of women aged 40 years and older who have received a mammogram within the preceding 2 years.
14. Increase the number of States that have a statewide population-based cancer registry that captures case information on at least 95 percent of the expected number of reportable cancers.
15. Increase the proportion of cancer survivors who are living 5 years or longer after diagnosis.

Source: http://www.healthypeople.gov/document/Word/Volume1/03Cancer.doc

www.ingramcontent.com/pod-product-compliance
Lightning Source LLC
Chambersburg PA
CBHW081834170526
45167CB00007B/2799